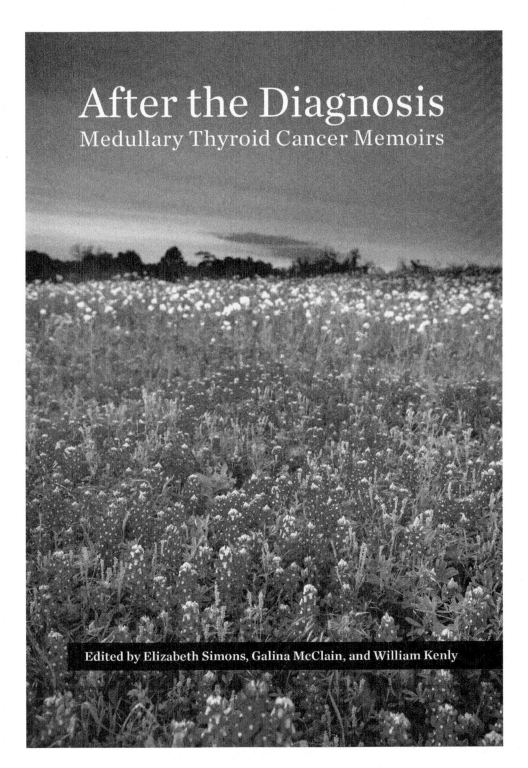

After the Diagnosis
Medullary Thyroid Cancer Memoirs

Edited by Elizabeth Simons, Galina McClain, and William Kenly

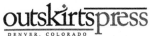

DENVER, COLORADO

The opinions expressed in this manuscript are solely the opinions of the author and do not represent the opinions or thoughts of the publisher. The author has represented and warranted full ownership and/or legal right to publish all the materials in this book.

After The Diagnosis, Medullary Thyroid Cancer Memoirs
All Rights Reserved.
Copyright © 2015 William Kenly
v2.0

Cover Photo © 2015 William Kenly. All rights reserved - used with permission.

This book may not be reproduced, transmitted, or stored in whole or in part by any means, including graphic, electronic, or mechanical without the express written consent of the publisher except in the case of brief quotations embodied in critical articles and reviews.

Outskirts Press, Inc.
http://www.outskirtspress.com

Paperback ISBN: 978-1-4787-6128-0
Hardback ISBN: 978-1-4787-6284-3

Outskirts Press and the "OP" logo are trademarks belonging to Outskirts Press, Inc.

PRINTED IN THE UNITED STATES OF AMERICA

Dedication and Acknowledgments

This book is dedicated to our Medullary Thyroid Cancer (MTC) "Meddie Stars" who have passed on, and several of their writings are included here. We have not highlighted them or put a notation by their names, because that would separate them, and they will forever be a part of us. They got their name "Meddie Stars" because of a tradition started a few years ago of going outside in the night when one of us had passed, and looking up and perhaps dancing, knowing that the heavens had one new star to watch over us.

The photography on the cover of this book is, "Vivid Bluebonnet Sunset" by Rob Bohning (www.RobBohningPhotography.com), with permission of Lori Bohning. Rob is a "Meddie Star" and was on his way back from treatment at MD Anderson to his family when he stopped his car and captured this scene.

Several others have contributed their time and efforts to make this a strong book. Myrtle Young spent weeks collecting the writings of the "Meddie Stars" and then the releases from those families.

The cover of this book was designed by John McClain. Legal consultation was provided by John-Henry Steele.

The initial printing of paperback copies offered through ThyCa were produced and donated by Dwight Vicks, the voluntary treasurer of the International Thyroid Oncology Group (ITOG), which collaborates to identify new treatments for advanced thyroid cancer, and can be contacted at www.ITOG.org. The entire proceeds from the sale of these copies go to MTC research. The royalties from the books bought through Amazon also go exclusively to ThyCa for research.

The Editors.

Table of Contents

Enjoy The Minutes You Have 1
By Elizabeth Simons

Rob 6
By Lori Bohning

Enjoy The Minutes You Have 11
By Jo-Anne Mauratt

New Life, New Normal 19
By Andrea Shelbourn

My Medullary Thyroid Cancer Story 24
By Lori Merritt

Lori's Husband Greg And His Story 30
By Greg

Lori's Mom Janet And Her Story 31
By Janet

Lori's Son Ryan And His Story 34
By Ryan

Three Camels, A Water Buffalo, And A Donkey With A Stroke 36
By Carol A. Corbitt

Circles 42
By Tamy Moretz

Inner Voice 44
By Joyce Johnson

Em Tough, Fight Like A Girl 46
By Hope Koehler

My MEN IIB Story 56
By Elizabeth Eastburn

Medullary Thyroid Cancer: Story Of Miracles 59
By Virginia Skilton

Support Is Crucial 69
By Vickie Baggett

Cancer Changes The Meanings Of Four Words 71
By William Kenly

Scared 77
By Anonymous

A True Oxymoron That Comes With Cancer 78
By Elizabeth Carey

I'm Still Here 88
By Michelle Wiley

The Long And Winding Road 92
By Elizabeth Simons

My Thank You Note To Cancer 96
By Joyce Johnson

One More Day With You 98
By Ashley Maderr

All The Signs 100
By Anna Johnson

Medullary Thyroid Cancer Is Not A Blessing 106
By Dara Michelle Hoffman

How Cancer Upended My Life—And Gave Rise To A New One 109
By David Kalish

Running Rampant 118
By Joyce Johnson

Listen To Those Inner Voices 123
By Karen Christianson

Take It Day By Day 129
By Terri Passanesi

My Body's Betrayal 132
By Mahaut de la Mare

What Cause Would Be Taking Up My Time? 134
By Kathryn Brubaker Wall

When You Get A Second Cancer 139
By Kathryn Brubaker Wall

The Squirrelly Kind Of Cancer 142
By Tami Weaver

The Diagnosis 144
By Sue Evert

Living With MTC 149
By Sue Evert

One Thing To Be Happy About 154
By Jo Gorringe

Dancing Through Cancer 156
By Jo Gorringe

Keeping It All In Perspective 158
By Bill Prentice

Remember To Take Care Of Yourself 162
By Becca

Obsession With Uncertainty 165
By Kerri Remmel

Diarrhea – The BIG D 168
By J. Doe

The "Big D" 170
By Bill Prentice

The Chosen One 174
By Joyce Johnson

Relearning How To Hope 177
By HJC

A Caregiver's Journal: In Rare Meddie Form 181
By Debbie Bambenek

A Mom's Journey With MTC 188
By Sharon Ferraro

Damn You, Cancer! 194
By Mary Belisle

A Day In The Life Of… 198
By Holly Bechard

When I Heard The Word Cancer 201
By Rae Charles

Meddie Memoir 212
By Myrtle L. Young

The Insidious Lump 218
By Karen Dewey

Waiting For The Waterfall 222
By ToniAnne Murray

I Realize How Short Life Can Be 226
By Becky Post

I Would Love To Think This Was Over **232**
By Elba Rosa Rodriguez

Carpe Diem! **234**
By Patty Dabrowski

Grateful And Lucky **236**
By Marion Sintenie

A Lightbulb Moment **241**
By Kristin MacFarland

Cancer Blows, Except When It Helps **243**
By Marilyn Geer Rivera

Find Joy In The Journey **245**
By Carolyn Willis

A Wild Ride **246**
By Anita Wright

Stand Up Straight And Keep Smiling **249**
Anonymous

Sonia And Marc **251**
By Sonia Prud'homme

We're Not Done Yet! **252**
By Virginia Skilton

Six Postings **260**
By Rob Bohning

Joni's Journey 265
By Joni Eskenazi

Five Generations 269
By Teresa Fountain

My MTC Journey 279
By Lois Godby

Today Is A Good Day For A Good Day 283
By Tammy Vetter

Life Without Parole: A Story Of Life With MTC 286
By Ralph Valeri

You're Screwed 293
By Karen Tesauro

Four Years And Counting 296
By Don Olson

How Did I Get This Cancer? 303
By Stanley Johnson

My Own Roller Coaster Ride 305
By Jan Hofer

The Dissection Of Thoughts 310
By Laura Druțău

Medullary Thyroid Cancer/MEN 2a, A Daughter's Story 315
By Christine S.

MTC: A Sister's Journey 318
By Lisa Leesman

It's The Small Things In Life That Count 320
By Mary Ann

Eager To Live 324
By Becky Mack

Diane's Story 328
By Diane Saxon

Bound Me Now To The Soil 332
By T. F. Tritt

Life Is Good And My Journey Continues 333
By Jan Hofer

Facebook Postings 338
By Julie Tavernier DiSanto

God Is Greater Than Any Problem I Have 339
By Tom Joiner

I Want To Be Well 345
By Christen Bordenkircher

Dear Cancer 355
By Megan Morrow Bozeman 355

Introduction

It was late one February evening during the Boston winter of 2015 when this idea, conceived of many minds, took root.

Sitting at my desk, trying to endure the fourth weekly one-foot-plus blizzard of the year, I was spending far too much time on Facebook. There was discussion in a group called "Medullary Thyroid Cancer-MTC" when Dave K. suggested we take all our stories and wrap them into a collection and publish it so others could benefit.

A firestorm of postings ensued. And slowly, over the next months, this book emerged.

The newbie meddies, several each week being introduced by Polly, were our original target audience. But then someone suggested that *anyone* fighting *any* cancer, or helping others to fight it, would benefit from this collection, because these stories are not so much about the details unique to MTC as they are about the psychological, emotional, family, and non-medical issues. Someone else chimed in to say that it is not just the cancer patients and caregivers who will benefit, but the doctors who treat cancer patients, the families of cancer patients, and the many others touched by cancer who could benefit from the understanding contained in these pages.

Another made the point that the real definition of "meddie" is not just the MTC veteran, but equally it is the caregiver, so that is how the term will be used in this book.

Here are a few terms that are not common in the non-meddie world:

- **Calcitonin and CEA** – Two blood markers for MTC. Calcitonin is unique to MTC, while CEA may come from other sources also. When trended over time, these hold meaning, both together and separately.
- **Dissection** – A long operation after diagnosis that attempts to remove most or all of the lymph nodes on one or both sides of the neck. A good doctor will diagnose the MTC before the total thyroidectomy (TT) and will do the TT and the Dissection together.
- **Endo** – Endocrinologist. This is the doctor who will follow you in the years ahead and adjust your thyroid medications. Only one doctor on your team needs to be an MTC expert, but that expert needs to have the experience of treating many meddies each week.
- **FNA** – Stands for fine needle aspiration, which is a biopsy done to determine pathology. A tissue sample is extracted from one or more lymph nodes using a very small needle the size of acupuncture needles.
- **Meddie** – A person, or their caregiver, who has Medullary Thyroid Cancer (MTC), an incurable, often inoperable, aggressive form of thyroid cancer.
- **PCP** – Primary Care Physician.
- **RET** – An acronym that stands for "rearranged during transfection." A test every meddie needs after MTC diagnosis to determine whether this is the hereditary form or the sporadic form of MTC.
- **Sporadic** – The non-inherited form of MTC, accounting for about 75 percent of all MTC.
- **ThyCa** – A world-wide non-profit organization dedicated to the support, education, and communication for thyroid

cancer survivors, their families and friends (www.ThyCa.org). All proceeds of this book go to ThyCa.
- **TKI** – A tyrosine-kinase inhibitor is a promising family of anti-cancer drugs. A pharmaceutical drug that inhibits tyrosine kinases, typically used as anti-cancer drugs.
- **TSH** – Thyroid Stimulating Hormone. The hormone produced in the pituitary gland that helps the thyroid function.
- **TT** – Total Thyroidectomy, a surgery that removes the entire thyroid.

For the new meddie, there are several sources of information:
- The "Revised American Thyroid Association Guidelines for the Management of Medullary Thyroid Carcinoma." Google it, read it, print it, and ask your doctor if he or she follows it. Only under extreme caution should you allow variations of these guidelines to be used on you. The Guidelines were written by the world-wide MTC experts.
- There are excellent Facebook MTC groups, and at least one Yahoo! group. There are several other Facebook groups for Multiple Endocrine Dysplasia (MEN). Join a few and read 100 or 1,000 posts. Ask questions. These are the meddie veterans (or survivors or warriors; everyone prefers a different moniker) who have walked this path, and its screwy side trails, for years, often decades.
- Every year ThyCa hosts a conference in a different city, usually in October. Many of the leading thyroid cancer doctors attend and lead sessions. When you attend, your understanding will take a huge leap. More importantly, you will discover that *you are not alone*. Since meddies make up only 1-2 percent of all thyroid cancer patients, meddies decided to wear Hawaiian shirts at last year's Conference so we could pick out other meddies in any

room. The rooms were flooded with Hawaiian shirts. You are *not* alone.

- There are two Amazon books about living with MTC, "The Opposite of Everything" by David Kalish, and "The Dogs of Cancer, Dancing with Medullary Thyroid Cancer" by William Kenly. Both bring this unusual cancer down a bit, to everyday understanding. "After The Diagnosis, Medullary Thyroid Cancer Memoirs" is the third book and it contains 84 personal stories from 66 meddies.

A few <u>Meddie Rules</u> to keep in mind:

- The "Meddie's Prime Directive": Get under the care of a doctor who treats several MTC patients every week. No other rule comes close to this imperative.
- Drive Your Own Bus: You are the final word on any treatment. If a medical professional tells you something that you do not agree with, even if it is said quite authoritatively, *you* make the decision.
- You Are Not Alone: 40% of people will hear a cancer diagnosis in their lifetime. One percent of all cancers are thyroid. One to two percent of thyroid cancers are MTC. If it weren't for Facebook and Yahoo!, none of us might ever meet another meddie. There is an army of meddies connected now.
- To A Man With A Hammer, Everything Looks Like a Nail. Doctors are not trained to heal all of you, they are trained to apply whatever discipline they have been trained in. A surgeon cuts. An oncologist uses radiation and chemotherapy. An internist prescribes pills. But who ties it all together? You do. See the second rule above.
- MTC Is Unlike Any Other Cancer. It presents itself, metastasizes, and is treated unlike any other cancer. It spreads

early and microscopically, so by the time it presents, it usually has spread outside the thyroid.

- When a meddie dies (*never* say, "loses her battle with cancer", no meddie is a 'loser'), we put on our Hawaiian shirts and go outside and look at our new meddie star up in the heavens. Some of us dance under that new star. We do this far too often. We hope our children will do it rarely. The proceeds of this book are going to support MTC research through ThyCa to make that hope come true.

- In the beginning of your journey, if any doctor uses the words "cure" or "iodine pills" or "chemo", you need to find another doctor. If any doctor says, "I will consult with the experts when we need to," or if any doctor tries to camouflage their lack of MTC experience by saying, "I treat many thyroid patients every week" or "I have been treating thyroid cancer for thirty years," stand up and leave. You need a doctor who treats several *MTC* patients every week. See the first rule above. More than 90 percent of meddies have had more surgeries than necessary because we started with a non-MTC expert. Don't have an unnecessary surgery.

Please register your thoughts about this book in a review on Amazon.com.

To contact the editors, write to: AfterTheDiagnosisMTC@gmail.com.

Thank you from your editors, Elizabeth Simons, Galina McClain, and William Kenly.

Standing In The Doorway

By Elizabeth Simons

I stand in the doorway, on the threshold of a luminous spring day, watching a paradise of birds swarm the feeder. The slanting light tells me it's nearing sunset, but it's still bright enough to see the iridescent cardinals, finches and woodpeckers feeding in the sunlight. I watch my husband round the corner on his lawn tractor, a knight if there ever was one, on a steed of fire and smoke, master of this world of birds and burgeoning flowers.

It is perfect, all of it, and all of it is fleeting. I can no more hold on to this picture than I can grasp a handful of water. We're told to seize the day. Be mindful. Live life to the fullest. As I stand in the fading sunlight with all this beauty before me, I don't know how much more I can be, how much more I can hold.

Can fullness be measured? Can it be more than it is? Is there any way I can make this last? Stop time and imprint the image on my heart? Is it possible to remain in this state of being forever? And most importantly, continue to be who I am in the process?

What will happen when I die? Will I enter a world parallel to this one? Will I remember these birds, this sunset, my husband, the children and grandchildren I love? The worst thing that could happen would be to cross the threshold and stop being me, with all my memories and experiences. How did this journey begin, and how will it play out in the theater of my soul?

I turn and go back into the house. The luminous moment dissolves. There is a meal to be prepared. A floor to be swept. As I chop vegetables, my attention wanders to the mundane.

The world quit being safe when I learned I had a cluster of cells that were behaving badly, growing where they shouldn't. Profligate cells multiplying their way around the isthmus between head and chest, holding my thyroid hostage until the only logical defense was taking it out.

It was then I first heard the word "cancer", spoken in hushed tones. Not just any cancer, but a particularly rare one, not treatable by conventional means. I learned it would be my dance partner for life, as there is no cure. Its manifestation would sometimes be courtly, sometimes rapacious. Its name was medullary.

My new reality plunged me into a maelstrom of denial. Cancer? I barred the door and held the word at bay. Too late. It was already inside.

Those who have cancer are often referred to as warriors. But I am no conquering heroine standing in a battlefield with the shards of cancer lying vanquished at my feet. I'm definitely not combative. I avoid conflict at all cost. Am I a warrior? Where's the battle? What am I fighting?

And whether I'm brave or cowardly, I still have cancer.

I find others online who have also received invitations to this medullary dance. Some, like me, have no symptoms other than relentless fatigue, while others are engaged in a constant struggle with a more aggressive cancer that devours internal organs like Pac Man's ghosts.

I feel overwhelmed and isolated. To begin with, I'm new to this support group and haven't had any long term contact with anyone. Other than cancer, we don't have shared experiences. Were it not for this St. Vitus' dance, we would not have met. How many times and in how many ways can I recite my fears? How many ways can I offer comfort to others whom I feel need more than I can give in the way of encouragement, especially when my own world is still so newly minted?

It's an immutable journey on a road with steep curves and no shoulders.

And while my fellow Meddies comprise a voluble partnership of cancer survivors through shared experiences, offering advice, insight and helpful information, I discover that family and friends are largely silent. I want to tell them, "This is what I'm going through. I don't understand much of what's going on, but I'll tell you what I know". Or, "I can steer you towards further information, if you want."

Amazingly, they don't want. Whenever I try to explain something to a friend or family member—such as why I'm tired all the time, or why surgery is often the only option for this type of cancer—the words bounce off a wall of silence. I'm puzzled. And hurt. Do they think my cancer is contagious? Does my demeanor suggest the kind of whiney self-pity that needs containment?

I begin to feel guilty. Had I been such a bad parent and spouse that my family should ignore me? Years earlier I had suffered depression and spent time in a hospital, which had required being away from family, both physically and emotionally, for an extended period. Were my children damaged by my absence and now must sanction me for my chaotic parenting?

Ironically, I'd thought then that I wanted to die. But something inside wouldn't let go. Something said to give it a chance. I might not have been the best parent or friend, but I did the best I could at the time, and when the chips were down, what I had to offer was faith. Faith that there was something bigger than this narrow world I had created, faith that even when all seemed hopeless, I had to trust otherwise.

And so it came to be that despite the bleak landscape in my soul, I climbed up and out of that black hole and emerged fully among the living. Was my legacy of triumph over self-destruction now overshadowed by this new threat of death?

I push irrational thoughts aside. First, death is inevitable. If not cancer, something else will take me. We all pray to die peacefully in our sleep, but life offers different scenarios. I'd like some insight into what lies ahead, come to terms with what it means to live in a world that I feel interpenetrates this one. How do I stay awake after I've crossed the threshold?

Because I believe that family and friends care about me, I resist the temptation to feel sorry for myself.

Perhaps they've just discovered the 800-pound elephant in the room, and it's threatening. Best to not look. Hadn't I always been the strong one? Hadn't I gone through life taking care of the needs of others? Hadn't I been the one who never asked for help because I saw it as a sign of weakness? Because I'm not displaying the usual cancer symptoms that come with radiation and chemotherapy, I appear to be healthy. Must I continue the exhausting role of being strong?

Years ago I was with my father as he lay dying. While he was able to speak he told me he knew it was his time, and he was at peace. Then he recited a story about when I was a little girl gathering eggs, clutching the basket to my chest and declaring that there were many more eggs in the hen house, but this was all I could carry.

My heart seized up. I held his hand and waited for more. I wanted words of wisdom, a final insight into how he'd managed to embrace life despite all the hardships he had endured, not some silly story from the past. But these were his last words.

Not long ago my son came to visit with his twin five-year-old boys. The kids played outside in the early spring weather while I watched from the sidelines. They were so full of life, so exuberant. Then one of the little guys came up to me and said, "Grandma, are you alright?" I assured him I was. When they were getting ready to leave, my usually reserved son said he was going to give me another hug before he left. And he did.

And then I knew.

Not all language is spoken. We don't always hear what we expect to hear. Why should I assume my father or my son would communicate differently? My father's last words were an act of love. He preferred acting to speaking, and his story was a pictorial farewell. Its power would sustain me after he was gone. My five-year-old grandson knew what words to say, and his compassion opened my soul. My son's extra hug was his way of telling me he loved me, and I am still warmed by this gesture.

So when I need to talk about the problems I face with unsympathetic doctors, or tell someone I'm hurting today, or if I need a question answered, I consult with my meddie friends, who are always there for me with a ready answer, because they know what I'm going through. I am awed and thankful for their unflagging support.

I find myself looking beyond my own self-consciousness. I understand that even on my worst days I'm loved, and I don't need to carry this burden alone. Accepting love from others also allows me to be less rigid and more gentle with myself.

Having medullary as a dance partner comes with an agenda. I never ask, "Why me?" Because in some deep part of my being I know I have extended the invitation.

What, then, am I supposed to learn? What do I need to know? Perhaps it's that no matter what comes to me from the future, I'll embrace it without being overwhelmed.

Being mindful isn't being in a perpetual state of bliss. It's making hundreds of little choices throughout the day, every day, so I can be present. Little moments are as great as extravagant ones. I'm learning to open my heart and make time to enjoy something. When a friend asks me to go somewhere, the sweeping can wait. The takeaway here is to prioritize what's essential and what is not.

I can't conquer cancer. But I can live with it. I can say yes to everything. Yes to anxiety, and yes to love and peace. I can trust that I'm given everything I need for all the life I have.

In the end, I can nudge the cancer and tell it to move over. We're in this together, for the long haul. The enemy is not cancer.

It's fear.

Rob

By Lori Bohning

In 2011, Rob was diagnosed with Medullary Thyroid Cancer. My husband was one of those people who kept up with his doctor visits and always made sure his physicals were up to date. I remember him once telling me that his greatest fear was to be sick and not be able to take care of his family. He always thanked God for his health. Rob was an incredibly healthy and strong man. I was always amazed at his endurance; he was one of those "man of all men" kind of a guy. He was a former Marine and he lived life as a Marine. A warrior.

His diagnosis was a shock. I remember him kneeling down beside me and holding me, saying, "Lori, we are going to beat this". It was the first of the millions of times he would say those words to me. He knew I needed to keep hearing that from him. The words, "it's positive" seemed unreal, and we kept thinking we were going to just deal with it and then quickly get out of the storm. We thought the battle would be short and we'd get back to our life. Little did we know, we were entering into the most horrific battle we ever could have imagined. I am talking about suffering on ALL levels.

Rob took the news and literally plowed forward. We didn't have too much time to feel, which was secondary. We just needed to gear up and fight. We joined some on-line support groups and someone mentioned there was a ThyCa conference that weekend in Los Angeles. We drove through the night to make this very important conference. I was emotional and Rob was encouraged. He asked every question and talked to many people. He was encouraged that others were surviving. When we got home, I remember praying that night, "God, please give him the best care". That next day, we were able to switch his insurance, which meant that we were able to go to MD Anderson. We didn't have time to think, we just made the appointment and a few weeks later, we were on a plane.

I remember a few solid things from the beginning part of our battle. I remember Rob had these sunglasses that were broken. I asked him why he didn't buy new ones. He stopped and thought, and then said, "I guess I thought, why buy new ones if I am going to die". That day, we decided to put a stop to that type of thinking. We made a commitment to live life as though we didn't have anything stopping us. Live life as though Rob didn't have cancer. *He* was not the cancer and we weren't going to bow down to it. It might slow him down, but it would never win. Cancer was not going to sabotage our life. We were *not* going to give it a foothold.

Another thing I remember was asking the question, "why?" We noticed that every time we asked that question, it brought us down, into a downward spiral. Rob said to me, "Why *not* us?"

In a way that it was an honor to be going through this. We know that only through suffering brings a refinement. So we embraced it and held our head high. Not proudly, but in a way, that we felt honored and glorified God, to be able to empathize and maybe even help with others in the same battle. Because after all, life is not all about us.

I also remember finding myself not having a purpose. My future seemed uncertain and I lived for the here and now. Someone gave me some wonderful advice. She said, "Don't stop dreaming. Dream new dreams!" That's what we did from that day forward. We made plans, we spent time with friends, we got out (even when Rob's legs were wrapped in bandages!). We talked about our future, we did things together, and if we had to cancel because of health issues, so we just canceled. Toward the end of Rob's life, we still continued to dream, we had our conversations that would last for hours into the night and morning. We dreamed. We talked about the past, present, and future. Some days, all we had was our talks and I will cherish those forever. I brought our dreams to him, and the outside world to him, and I can still hear him say, "What else, Lori, what else happened?"

Something happens when you realize that your body in the mirror isn't what it once was. When you look and you are almost afraid to see who is looking back. A beautiful thing happens. You realize that life isn't what the world said it was, all the media, all the people with empty words. You realize that you have something that nobody else has and it's not the cancer. Not only have you met the most amazing people, friends that are real, but your soul has been lifted to a level that so many have never or will never experience. You realize it's so *not* about flesh and blood; it's about what is on the inside. It's the beauty of the battle that shines from inside. We learned more about humanity than any book could have taught us. We were able to put away the facade and reach out to others with an understanding. Anyone who knew Rob knows he was a straight shooter. He would cut right to the heart of the issue. No bull with Rob. He was real.

I fell more in love with Rob during those three and a half years, than I ever thought was possible. It's those times when you sit, knowing what is ahead, and just sit silently, hand in hand.

This is a part of what I wrote for Rob's Memorial:

> *"I know there was a point where Rob truly understood that his body was only a fleshly vessel, and it wasn't what all of us are here for. All of us who know God are set apart for a divine purpose. Yes, the beast of cancer ravenously destroyed his body, but it never once touched Rob's faith. We knew that the longer gold is in the refining fire, the more pure it becomes, the more it shines, and the more people are drawn to it. Cancer never won because we knew that if we had Christ,*

there would always be victory. So, God saw Rob's heart could be used, and no, it wasn't a lofty ministry. There was nothing glamorous about it. The mission field was a humble one with tremendous suffering, where your soul utterly falls in sheer helplessness at the feet of Jesus. Rob told me if this was the only thing he was called to do to honor God and bring glory to Him, then He wanted to do the job well. And he did, and God is SO pleased with my husband. My husband was not cancer. Rob was a wonderful husband, father, and friend. Rob sure did love his family! Never one day passed that we didn't know he loved us. He endured so much suffering to stay just another moment with us. By God's grace, he lived over three years with a very aggressive disease. He lived for his family and we adored him and loved him to pieces. He was everything to me."

We have two children. They were 4 and 6, when Rob was diagnosed. They have been a part of this battle since the day he was diagnosed. They didn't understand fully, and it was with a little education that they did understand what it meant to have cancer. Both children dealt with it differently. My son felt overwhelmingly helpless. He wanted to help his daddy and it killed him to see Rob in pain. He wanted to do something and help in some way to make it better for his daddy. So, he did a triathlon for MTC last June. My daughter, being younger, would rub Rob's back and bring him food. When Rob had to tell her he couldn't take her to the Valentine's Day dance, she stood up and put her hand on his shoulders and said, "It's ok, Daddy, I understand". They saw the face of suffering through all the needles, drains, scars, medicines, and they experienced it with Rob when he was not able to participate in things, or when he had to leave early because of the effects of the medicines. They saw the nurses come and go, and they heard conversations between adults about Rob's condition. Rob told them throughout the cancer battle to never give up, keep praying, and to stand strong. Always. They saw a warrior in action and it will be with their souls forever. They saw his faith that never wavered. They saw a silent warrior, never complaining, just fighting with each breath simply because he loved his family.

Enjoy The Minutes You Have

By Jo-Anne Mauratt

You have cancer. But don't worry, it's a mixture of papillary and follicular cancer. While the specialist kept talking, she lost me at "you have cancer". That was 14 years ago.

I've been blessed with having the same family physician for more than 26 years. When I went to her stating that the doctor I worked for noticed a lump in my neck, she immediately sent me for tests and referred me to a specialist. By that time, I knew if Rose was worried there was a good reason for it.

It was a few months before I met with the surgeon. I had a biopsy done and went to her office for the results. The specialist was quick and to the point, "So, you have cancer. We'll go in and remove it and give you radioactive iodine. Don't worry, you're lucky. You have the 'good' cancer!"

What? There's a *good* cancer? I had worked more than 15 years in the medical field and had never heard someone describe cancer that way.

I went home and told my family, "Don't worry, it's the good kind." At the time I was recently separated and had four children living at home. I read everything I could find on the type of cancer I had and felt better. After all, it was better than the other two types of thyroid cancer.

On my 38th birthday I had my thyroid removed. The surgery went well and afterwards my son said I resembled Frankenstein's monster.

The specialist told me the surgery was a success and the cancer had not spread outside the thyroid. She explained that there was a 20-year survival rate for people who had this type of cancer and were untreated. I felt relieved. I'd been worried for nothing. Life went on.

A few years later, in 2004, I started having dizzy spells, night sweats and issues with my blood pressure. All the tests led up to the fact that I had a pheochromocytoma, a rare tumor that starts in the cells of your adrenal glands. I had a number of tests done and an endocrinologist sent me for genetic testing.

After testing in the genetic department of our local children's hospital, I was called in for the results and was shocked when I was told I had Multiple Endocrine Neoplasia (MEN) IIa. They explained that this was a genetic condition that caused thyroid cancer as well as pheochromocytoma. I was then asked to bring in my children for testing.

My oldest daughter tested first, as she was thinking of starting a family. My two youngest were willing to have the test, but my oldest son did not want it.

It was very hard on me to think I might have given my children a disease where they could get cancer, even if it was the "good" cancer. What parent does that? I cried for days and said a lot of prayers. The day came for the results and we found out only my oldest son carried the gene. My heart broke. What did this mean for him? Would his children get it?

My specialist was not receptive to me having an adrenalectomy. When I informed her I had MEN IIA she stated she had figured that out years ago. I was angry. How could she not have told me? If there were other surgeons who could have done the surgery, I would have changed doctors.

I was booked and went to the hospital prior to the day of surgery. The day of the surgery came and I was taken down to the OR. No matter how many surgeries I've had, that horrible feeling of being strapped to a cold table surrounded by light and instruments is never good.

When I entered the hospital I was told my surgery would be two small incisions in my back. I woke up naked and intubated in the intensive care unit. It seemed that something had gone wrong and I'd required an incision from one side of my stomach to the other. I was having trouble breathing and needed oxygen. I spent weeks in the hospital and months at home recuperating. I could hardly move, and sitting up was exhausting. My family was afraid something would happen to me. It was a long recuperation. However, I was lucky, as I had short term disability to help with the finances.

When my son went to a surgeon to have his thyroid removed, he refused to go see the same one I had. He'd had a thyroidectomy when he was 27. Unfortunately, by that time he had cancer. When they took out his thyroid they stated that they got it all.

When I think back to that time, I felt like I was losing my mind. After the surgery I had no control over my emotions. I could go from happy to crying to anger in three seconds or less. PMS looked good by comparison. I was horrible to live with. I either ate too much or too little. I had no energy and was not sure I'd survive.

Try doing all that with a smile on your face and pretending life is great. My older daughter and I now joke about how many times she had "talked me off the ledge."

Like everything in life, time helps you accept what you can't change. I went on with my daily life and tried to make the best of things. I was sad that my wonderful son's personality changed from a happy-go-lucky to very quiet. I think watching the change in him was worse than anything. Although his medical issues were stable, his smile was gone.

I thought life with MEN IIa wasn't so bad. I was learning to live being steroid dependent, going to the hospital for common colds, the shots, the medications. Then in 2013 I was in a car accident. In the ER the doctor told me my ribs were fine, but the cancer in my lungs had spread. *Cancer in my lungs?* What the hell was he talking about? I told him that was the first I'd heard about this.

He gave me a requisition for a CT scan. After the scan I had a neck ultrasound. After that I had a fine needle biopsy of the nodules they found in my neck. Within days I found out I had Medullary Thyroid Cancer (MTC). I thought to myself, "Okay, I was told I had the good cancer, so how did it spread? Maybe I was exaggerating things." Then I read what Medullary Thyroid Cancer was. No treatment per se, terminal, life expectancy of less than 10 years for 20-40 percent of people whose cancer had spread outside the thyroid. Wait! Mine hadn't spread or at least it hadn't been confirmed, or so I told myself, totally disregarding the neck biopsy.

I was scheduled to see a respirologist, who booked me for a bronchoscopy. Within days of the procedure I found myself sitting in the specialist's office with my oldest daughter as we received the news that I had mastic medullary cancer, which was now in my lungs.

I remember leaving the office and trying not to be upset. My daughter asked me if I was okay. "Sure," I lied, but a few tears escaped. I don't think she believed me. I held it together until I got in my car. Then I turned up Reba and cried all the way home.

I'd had this cancer from 2000. How could I tell my kids it was back and would only get worse? I asked my oldest not to tell the others until I could tell them myself. At this point they knew something was up. How could I tell my older son, who had already gone through so much, that I'd been wrong? He couldn't look at me and see everything would be okay. That if I wasn't sick, he wouldn't be, either, when in fact he might end up with cancer in the long term. In the end my daughter told them. I couldn't.

My daughter and I went to see the local oncologist. We don't have a specialist who deals specifically with MTC. He told me that chemotherapy and radiation were not an option, adding that there were medications to help with "end stage" cancer. However, they weren't a cure, but were given to help slow progression, and might make me more ill. There were some drug trials, but for now it was sit and wait.

I left the office thinking, "I had a new grandson, only one child was married, and two were still in college. Would I see them get through later milestones? Would I see my son buy a house and have children?

Would I die alone? Would my grandson remember me? Would it hurt? How long would I live?" These and a thousand other questions ran through my head. I had spent my whole live being strong, independent, and trying to handle everything myself. How could I pull this one off?

I went online and found a great group and heard about a conference in Philadelphia. My daughter and son-in-law paid for my trip to Philly to find out more information. The people I met there were amazing. Everyone was very helpful and informative. I learned so much that when I returned home a little of that initial fear had gone away.

I knew that over the years since my adrenalectomy my health had suffered. I'd lost a kidney, had trouble sleeping, my immune system was so compromised it took only a day for me to catch the bug. I can't count the number of times I've visited the emergency room. I was cold one minute and hot the next. I took a trip and I was tired. I couldn't walk or do as much as I used to. However, I'd told myself "It's okay. You're getting old!" Now what would I tell myself? How would I stay positive?

For the last two years I'd gone through life trying to live it the best I could. I have good times where I have lots of energy and other times where doing the dishes seems like a major chore. Some days even getting out of bed takes all my energy. I found something that I could get out of bed for. My grandson. My children are older and have their own lives. My grandson makes me laugh, smile, and look at life through his eyes. When he says, "You okay, Nana?" I know I'll be there for him.

Over the last year I've noticed changes to my health. I'm embarrassed that I clean my small condo in spurts. Some days it takes two hours to do the whole thing, other times it takes me a week to clean it, just in time to start over.

I have trouble breathing, and sometimes swallowing causes coughing spells, as do mornings going out in the cold. I wonder if I'm still going up the hill, on top of it, or heading down the other side.

I changed to a less stressful job last year. I joined a wonderful online group that makes me laugh. I think of a lady name Joy who dances on tables, and I laugh! I read all the comments, yet don't post much. Just reading helps, and the education they supply is priceless. It helps, as they understand what others cannot.

In Canada we don't have the medical expertise they do in the United States. While free health care is great, the knowledge would be just as great. I've learned to laugh at myself, and to do things I would never have done if not for the cancer, so maybe it is a blessing in disguise.

I keep telling myself:

    a) The world won't stop if you can't do the dishes until tomorrow.

    b) Travel now, later might never come.

    c) Take the time to be with your family, because one day your time will run out.

    d) Enjoy the minutes you have. Or better yet, make them.

    e) Don't worry about schedules. Cancer doesn't have one.

Yes, I still cry, only not as much. At times I get upset and do things I probably should not have done. I now spend as much time as I can with my children and my two wonderful grandsons. I choose to spend time enjoying them, doing things with them and taking things one day at a time. I choose the good things.

For me the medical side of things is scary. I can live with scary. The emotional side is much harder!

When I look around the play center, I look like every other Nana there. Only I know I'm different. I know that I'll probably not see my grandsons grow up. I most likely won't see them finish elementary school, let along high school. I wonder, "Will Kai's hair stay red? Will Nico develop his daddy's personality? How will they do in school? Will they take after their mommy?" I take so many pictures, hoping with each "click" that they'll remember the time we spent together, even if they forget about me.

I can't change my health, so I choose to take each day as it comes.

I see my grandsons now, I hug them, play with them and make memories with them now. It's not easy, but I try.

It's a great comfort to know that if I don't get to attend that graduation, or wedding, or birth, that part of me will be there. The part of me that lives in each one of my children.

Each day brings different things to handle. On our recent trip to Disneyland, I was so disappointed that I couldn't keep up with my family. They were great, because they never expected me to. I was embarrassed that I couldn't walk as far. I was tired, hot, and felt I was holding them back. At one point I got upset with my son-in-law because he was trying to be helpful. I felt useless, yet he would never make me feel that way. It's hard to lose independence.

I know that people are generally concerned, and that makes life easier. Some people don't realize that some of the comments they make are upsetting. Why do you have a handicapped sticker? You look fine. If I explain I have thyroid cancer and some days are not good days, I hear, "Oh, you have the good cancer." I ask them how is it good to live with a ticking time bomb that will change your whole family's lives? How is it good to know you'll have to suffer pain, indignity, financial hardship, loneliness and death? How is it good to look at your family and know you're dying, yet don't know when?

Through this whole process the hardest part for me is that every day I see that I'm losing the one thing I have held in high esteem: my independence. I've gone through the embarrassment of many medical personnel seeing me naked, not being able to keep up with people my age, and having to use a mobile device to get around.

Just recently I had another ultrasound and found out the cancer has spread. I'm being referred back to a specialist and may possibly have another surgery. Deep down my doctor and I know I'm not a candidate for surgery. The look on her face tells me it's the beginning of the end. Yet I keep the faith. However, my family is scared, and I've learned that this is also their journey. Making them happy and comfortable is something I can do, so I do what I can.

Just in case, my family moved up a trip to Hawaii. Even though I wish we didn't have to, we seem to live life on a schedule that revolves around my illness. My son-in-law is wonderful for being so patient and caring, as are all my children.

It's hard to be hopeful when there doesn't seem to be any hope. It's hard to stay positive all the time. So we take one day and one step at a time, and hope that each step will last years.

So for Joyous, for making me laugh at your adventures and the fact I don't have the "Big "D," for Carol, for keeping me informed on the latest information, for Polly, for just saying hi, and for rest of the group for telling their stories, giving me answers to medical questions and being there, I thank you. Oh, and I forget Bill, for making me hungry in the middle of the night so I am off to make a grilled cheese and turkey bacon sandwich that will keep me awake the rest of the night. But it'll be worth it!

Each one of us Meddies is different, yet we're similar in many ways. We do the best we can and take one day at a time. On our online site we've learned to rely on each other. It makes us laugh and shows us there's hope, even when it seems otherwise.

New Life, New Normal

By Andrea Shelbourn

"It's bad news I'm afraid…You have thyroid cancer." Those were the words that came tumbling out of the consultant's mouth. Strangely, it didn't come as the massive shock you might imagine to this 41 years old.

Almost 5 years previous, I had gone to the doctor's with a swollen lymph node in my neck. On examination, he had decided it was fine, and he instructed me to "keep an eye on it". I had mentioned it to several other doctors over the 4 plus years that followed and all came to the same conclusion. "Nothing to worry about." So I didn't. I carried on with my life in the bliss of ignorance.

Then in the July of 2014 my lump was joined by a friend, a new lump. I went to visit a new doctor who was very thorough indeed, he did countless blood tests, but couldn't find anything wrong, so he decided to refer me to the hospital as he was all out of ideas! I met the first of many consultants. He too said it was nothing to worry about. The doctor and consultant did keep asking me about night sweats, weight loss and itching, I had none of these symptoms; in fact I felt just fine! I had a biopsy and an ultrasound done and when I got home I did what any doctor will tell you not to do, I started to google. Limited options for swollen lymph nodes, tends to be either cancer or infection, seeing as I'd had it 5 years, infection was unlikely so on googling including the night sweats, weight loss and itching, which I didn't have, I decided I had non-Hodgkin's lymphoma.

My reply to those immortal words "you have thyroid cancer" weren't those of breaking down in tears, or getting angry or an outpouring of emotion in any way really, but instead I calmly replied, "Oh, I haven't googled that!". He told me it was very rare and my treatment would take place in a specialist hospital in Oxford, about an hour's drive away and that was that. I walked out of the room with my husband Paul, hand in hand, in silence. I can't put into words my feelings at that point, just numb.

My whole life's plan had changed in an instant. I was about to embark on the biggest fight of my life, I was entering a world of the unknown.

And I didn't like it.

When my two gorgeous boys came in from school, Ben, aged 14 at the time, and Thomas, aged 12, we told them straight away. We've always been a close-knit family unit, we've never had secrets, and everything has always been honest and open. They were unsurprisingly upset and we all had a good cry. We decided to call the tumour Bernard, just seemed like a more light hearted way to talk about this very serious matter. I think that for me, this was one of the few times I have cried (except actually whilst writing this! I've been blubbing the whole time whilst I've been typing this. I guess that proves it comes straight from the heart). You may be misled at this point to thinking I am naturally quite an unemotional person where as in fact I'm the opposite. I've always liked a good cry. I never miss an opportunity! But somehow this situation was different, I almost felt like crying was like letting Bernard win and I certainly am not going down without a fight!

Thomas is very open with his thoughts and emotions and his first question was, "Are you going to die?" I replied that I didn't intend on dying yet! But naturally, it has been a constant thought in my head, the possibilities of leaving my boys behind without a mummy and being denied the future I'd planned with Paul, all the things we were going to do and places we were going to visit as we grew old together. It just all seemed so unfair for all of us. I told my best friend via a text whilst still in the hospital. She isn't a touchy feely emotional person at all, but even she spent the afternoon crying. I decided after that to tell everyone by text, that way I didn't have to witness the crying or despair in their faces. I did stipulate on every text I didn't want pity or sympathy, as I've never got on well with it.

My doctor tried it once at the very beginning, I told him off! He's never done it again. I need facts not fluffiness! My family and friends were all amazing. I was incredibly well supported and felt so loved and cared for. I think Paul has probably felt the most helpless in all this, he was going through this huge rollercoaster of emotion with me and yet he was forgotten about whilst I sat firmly in the limelight. Through all this, he has been my rock, I could never ask for anything more, he's spent countless hours waiting whilst I've had scans and tests done, he never moans, just holds my hand and hugs me when it's over. Our endless love for each other alone will get us through this. He has asked the question, "Why you?" many times; to that there is no answer other than, "Why not me?" My dearest mum endured ovarian cancer at 52 and breast cancer at 75. I'm sure she never asked that question. She just accepted the hand life had dealt her and battled against it. Likewise my darling dad had a massive brain hemorrhage at 48. Next year, against all the odds they both will celebrate their 80th birthdays. My parents are my inspiration. I definitely come from a family of tough cookies.

I had a CT and an MRI scan and then went to see my new consultant in Oxford. He said it looked like it was all contained in my neck and hopefully they'd be able to remove it all and that would be that (If only!). I had my operation on the 23rd of January this year. Foolishly I'd googled it and wished I hadn't! Thomas had asked me the morning before, how many people a year die under general anesthesia? I said google it and tell me after, when I'm not one of the statistics! Although he also said he wanted my thyroid and Bernard brought home in a jar! The operation went ok although the findings were worse than my scan had shown. I ended up having my jugular removed (always thought it is a vital part of a neck, but evidently not!). A full thyroidectomy and radical neck dissection, I had 30 lymph nodes removed of which 16 were cancerous and my laryngeal nerve was cut and re-stitched. I'm due to start radiotherapy very soon, but the cancer has unfortunately also appeared on my spine, so as I'm writing this, I'm waiting to see what the next move after radiotherapy in this very complex treatment game is.

I was very lucky to have stumbled across my fellow "meddies" on Facebook, Medullary being so rare. Finding out anything about it is a challenge, let alone actually meeting someone who has it. They answered so many questions that I didn't even think of asking. It was a bit of a double edged sword though, one day I would read something really positive and I'd feel really upbeat, and then another day I'd read something much harder to take, like the passing of a fellow meddie, and I'd be catapulted into the pits of despair for a while.

This has certainly opened my eyes to what really matters. In life you just plod along getting on with things and then one day you realize you're old and the children have grown up and you haven't done all those things you were going to do. This has made me appreciate every single day with my amazing family.

So for the moment at least, I'm living this new life. A new normal. Not the care free one I'm used to. A cancer bubble if you like. A seemingly endless cycle of doctors' appointments, blood tests and scans. Every hospital appointment is like a rollercoaster, jump on board the anxiety train up to the appointment, then, depending on the news, misery or elation after. I've endured things that a few years ago I would never have believed possible, like having my radiotherapy mask fitted.

I am a much stronger person than I ever imagined I could be. The doctor warned me of "dark days". I think I've been lucky, as both Paul and I have had dark moments, but luckily not at the same time, and we have managed to snap each other out of it. At the end of the day, life's too short to waste any moments worrying about something that you can't change. I've heard the words, "You're so brave" quite a bit. One of my fellow cancer survivors said it was because people think in your situation they would never cope. But they would. You have to. There is no other choice. In the face of adversity you deal with whatever's thrown at you. Cancer is not going to break me. Cancer is not going to beat me.

All I can say is: "F**k you cancer, you chose to mess with the wrong girl! I WILL BEAT YOU!"

My Medullary Thyroid Cancer Story

By Lori Merritt

My name is Lori and I was 34 years old when I was diagnosed with Medullary Thyroid Cancer.

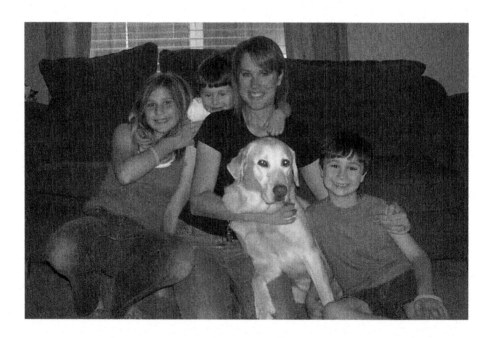

That day was in July 2004. A wife and a mother to an eight-year-old daughter, Kalie, four-year-old son, Nathan, and eight-month-old baby boy, Ryan. That day has forever changed my family and me. Shortly after being diagnosed with sporadic Medullary Thyroid Cancer, I had my total thyroidectomy surgery. Thank God I didn't have the hereditary type, my babies are safe. Post-surgery, was hell, my face and mouth felt droopy, and when I saw myself in the mirror! My gosh, my neck had a scar from ear to ear with staples all up and down my incision.

Looking back at my nine-hour surgery and week-long hospital stay, certain things really stuck out in my mind. I found out the doctors took eighty-three lymph nodes and twenty-four tested positive for MTC. During my surgery they almost couldn't save my vocal cords because most of the cancer was on or around them. And then the clincher! My doctor told me she estimated that I had seven years to live. I was stage 3 and there is no treatment for Medullary besides surgery. Then my doctor left my hospital room while I cried, and my mom walked in to see how I was doing. There was one happy memory during my stay, when all three of my kids came to visit me in the hospital and I went down to the entrance of the hospital to sit with my family. My baby Ryan took his very first steps in the hospital, so I got a little happiness out of that long week.

Coming home and adjusting to living with cancer was very hard for me, especially hearing from my doctor that I only had 7 years to live. That's all I could think about. Seeing my very young children and thinking of their future without their mother put me into a huge depression. I cried all the time. I wrote my children goodbye letters. I remember putting my two older children on their school buses and just crying after the bus left because I knew I wouldn't be there for their graduations and their futures. How could I leave my children? I can't think about that time again when all I could do was cry. I was helpless over cancer. Needless to say, I soon switched doctors to someone who had some sort of experience with MTC. I was also learning to live with cancer, and beginning to live again.

Two years after being diagnosed I found out that my cancer had metastasized to my shoulder. Weird I know, but it mentally freaked me out. Shortly after that my cancer metastasized to my spine and neck. I was so distraught, so upset. I had conflicting opinions from different doctors. I had radiation on my shoulder. My radiation doctor telling me MTC is slow growing you'll live a long life... breathe. Then I had my new doctor telling me that I won't grow old and see my children grow up because my cancer has metastasized and they can't treat it with surgery. Depression hit again... my main doctors gave me NO hope at all. This has happened twice for me with the horrible repercussion of their words. With my depression I so desperately needed hope, I needed to know there were others living with MTC. I sought out the Medullary Yahoo! support group. This is where I learned I was not alone, there were others living with MTC, others who had so much knowledge and strength. Through this group I found out about the ThyCa conference coming up in Baltimore. I knew I needed to go, I needed to meet others and hear their stories. My husband and I went and I met fellow MTC patients who have been living with cancer for 10, 20, 30 yrs. This was the hope I so desperately needed.

After this trip to Baltimore and finding the Medullary Yahoo! support group, I found a Facebook Medullary support group too. I slowly started gaining knowledge and started advocating for myself. I didn't look at my life anymore like I was dying of MTC, like two doctors had told me I was going to do. I knew I was in charge of my cancer journey, and I had the knowledge and strength now. I was learning to live my life with cancer and learning to be happy with it all.

My husband and I ended up separating in 2009 and divorcing in 2010. No, I don't think it had anything to do with the cancer, he was quite wonderful through everything cancer related. Later when I started dating is when it got weird. When do you tell someone new you have cancer? "Hi. I'm Lori, I have cancer?" No! First date? No, second date? Probably not. You want someone new to get to know you, not the cancer patient. I don't ever want to be defined by having cancer. Well, I don't at least. And when you do tell someone special you have cancer, it's awkward because you don't know if they will reject you. Or if their family will reject you? Or maybe you just don't want to subject anyone to the whole cancer world. It's a lot to take, it never ends, especially financially. When is the right time to tell a new person in your life?

"Who would ever want me, I'm a stage 4 cancer patient. My cancer bills will never end, my cancer appointments will never end, my cancer will never end." I kept telling myself. But I did start dating and all my fears came full force, but I was never rejected. Everyone I dated accepted my cancer, and no, I didn't tell them on the first date, it took a while. And that was ok.

Then I met my future husband, Greg. On our first date, Greg saw my scar on my neck. I had no choice but to tell him. It freaked me out because he was full of questions and all I wanted to do was talk about anything but cancer. I didn't want to talk about it, because I didn't want him to start seeing me as a cancer patient. All my fears aside, I tried to answer everything he asked about me. And that was on our first date. And guess what, it didn't scare him away! We got married a quick four months later!

After getting married, I found a great local doctor who gave me so much hope. I also started getting my check-ups at MD Anderson under Dr. Hu. Although it took me a while to form my medical team, now I'm secure and happy. I feel I've got the best medical team working for me. I've been on Caprelsa since February of 2012. Now three years later I'm stable. Mentally I know when Caprelsa stops working there are other options. Currently I have metastases to my spine and skull. My cancer seems to like my bones (hehehe). I started taking Caprelsa on 2/2012 and about a couple months later I noticed my hair was falling out and thinning out. The shock of Caprelsa to my body took a huge hit to my hair!! That was really hard for me. I had long hair and I didn't realize how much my hair meant to me as a woman. I've had long hair all my life and now I had to cut it all off. Before I cut my hair, I remember going to work and trying to hide my hair falling out by styling it differently. A coworker confronted me and I just started crying there at work. I knew it was time to cut off my hair. Another thing cancer was taking from me. Yes, I know hair will grow back, but I was angry. My long hair hid my scar, now having very short hair I had nothing to hide behind.

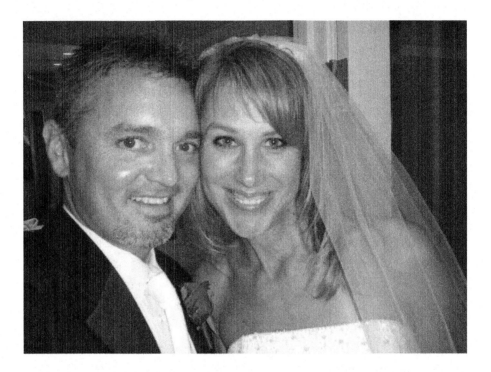

I sure am at a different spot than I was years ago. Yes I do have bad days, or bad weeks. I go through the rollercoaster of emotions. I know it's normal. This July will be eleven years living with cancer. I say it with a smile, I'm stronger now, and I'm a better advocate for myself and for others. I'm a better person because of my cancer journey.

My daughter Kalie was eight years old when I was diagnosed and I was told by two doctors I wouldn't be alive to see my children grow up. Guess what? I was a proud momma as I watched my daughter graduate from High School in 2014!!

I get to see my children grow up.

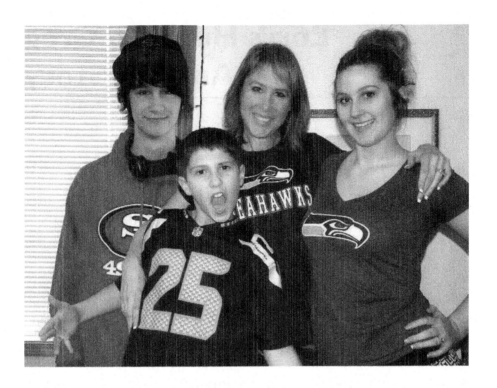

Cancer changes people. It sculpts us into someone
Who understands more deeply, Hurts more often, appreciates
More quickly, cries more easily, Hopes more desperately, loves
More openly, and lives more passionately.

Lori's Husband Greg And His Story

By Greg

Nobody slips through God's fingers. That is what I've always felt. God brought Lori into my life, and won't take her out till He is good and ready, which is good enough security for me. I trust that as long as we continue to be vigilant in our pursuit of treatment, things remain in His hands, though Lori wants to take control back sometimes. Lori and I have every opportunity to be happy on this Earth together just as any other couple. It's all in what we do with the time we're given.

Lori's Mom Janet And Her Story

By Janet

A Mother's Prayers

Dear God, I am praying. Please watch over my daughter, Lori, in her battle with Medullary Thyroid Cancer. Keep her strong, keep her safe, and take care of her worries. I am praying for the doctors who are treating her. I am praying for a cure for this horrendous form of cancer.

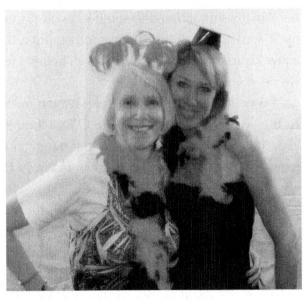

I have prayed for her in many cathedrals and churches in Italy and France, St. Peter's/Vatican, Notre Dame, Assisi, just to name a few.

I have lit a candle in Lourdes, France and prayed for her with tears running down my cheeks. This holy city, where pilgrims from around the world pray for a cure. What an honor to be able to do this in Lori's name!

Lori was a sweet and lovely child who became an adult woman with tenacity, stubbornness, and endurance. Where did she get these traits, I was soon to find out. A phone call from my daughter changed my life in 2004. She remarked that she had a swollen lymph node on the right side of her neck, which she had had for quite a while. I quickly grabbed my medical symptoms book. The book stated it could a simple virus - to lymphoma. We have no recent family history of cancer, but the "seed" had just been planted in my brain.

Mixed, heavy emotions hung over me the day she had her tumor biopsied. After the surgery, her doctor came out into the waiting room to inform Lori's husband any me that, "things don't look so good". What do you mean, I thought to myself, this is my daughter and this is all a nightmare. I held her husband's hand in the waiting room and prayed to God for a miracle. Numbed, shocked, trying to keep it all together, waiting to see her. I am her mother, so I have to keep a brave face for her. Finally I'm allowed to see her. I will never forget, she asked "why me"? A mother is supposed to protect, put a band aid over their hurts, a few kisses and hugs and make it all better. I felt powerless. Dear God, we need you!!

I was with Lori later while she waited for her big surgery to begin. As they were wheeling her to the O.R., I thought what do I do, what do I say. It was as if God said, "Put your daughter in my hands". I held her hand and said to her, "You are now in God's Hands." Little did I know how right I was!

Our family and friends gathered in the waiting room of the hospital while the surgery went on to remove her thyroid and numerous tumors. It was a very lengthy surgery, and finally her doctor came out and stated that it took over 2 1/2 hours to remove all the tumors surrounding her vocal cords. Further, she said, half way through the procedure some of the doctors wanted to sever the vocal cord to finish the job of removing the tumors. Praise God's answer to my prayers, the remaining physicians voted to keep working on her vocal cords, with a great outcome!

For months after the surgery, Lori was very angry at God, which is not unusual. I remember telling her to stop these negative feelings and accept God back into her life. So proud of her! Many months later, Lori, her daughter Kalie, and myself were baptized wearing our ThyCa pins. One of the greatest moments of my life.

Thus began a long journey of doctor's appointments, procedures, blood counts and travelling to various cities to see if she could qualify for the trial medications. She never saw me cry, never knew how I felt helpless as a mother, and never knew the emotional toll it took to keep going. All she saw was love, encouragement and faith that somehow it would be okay.

The remaining years have become somewhat of a blur. But I have come to understand why God gave her such tenacity, stubbornness and endurance. God made her the way she is so she could fight the fight of her lifetime, battling Medullary Thyroid Cancer. She is winning the fight… Thank You Lord!

Lori's Son Ryan And His Story

By Ryan

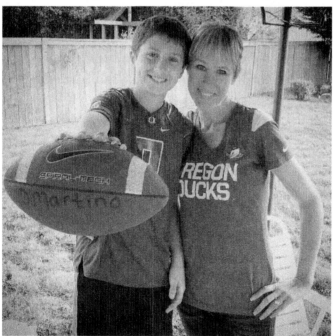

My name is Ryan. I am 11 years old and my mom has cancer. It affects me because my mom has to go to the hospital a lot and sometime she stays at the hospital for a long time. I remember when I was about 5 years old and my mom had radiation therapy. My Grandma had to come take care of us. When my mom came home she was all droopy and just not herself. My dad had to help her do lots of things. Finally after several months she started feeling herself again. This happened two times, my mom had radiation twice.

When my friends find out my mom has cancer they always say, "I'm sorry". I always say back "why?" If you don't have a parent or anybody you know who has cancer then you would think I am crazy for saying "why?" But I am not crazy, I am just used to it.

My mom having cancer can be scary sometimes because I always wonder if she might die from cancer. When my Mom had surgery on her back, my sister came home crying saying it was cancer related and that my Mom might die. I was sitting on my bed listening and was worrying about what would happen if my mom died. It is hard. It is harder than you think.

Every 6 months my mom travels to Texas to get her check up's, that part is hard too.

By Ryan (Lori's youngest child)

Three Camels, A Water Buffalo, And A Donkey With A Stroke

By Carol A. Corbitt

True life is always stranger than fiction. It can be fun or strange or stranger than strange, but it is always the basis for the best stories. My medullary journey has been no exception.

When looking to explain the "Who, What, Where, When or Why" of a *rare* disease, the average person has no reference for an unknown. Mortality itself is a life-long search for answers. For me, I look out the windows off my porch deck and gaze at the biggest example of medullary I can find. It's all in my pastures or a short drive to our little downtown.

Out of any window I can see Sebastian, Miko and Milo, the camels, grazing by the water buffalo, Dundee. The next pasture holds One-Eyed Jack, a mini donkey. He has had a stroke and thus the name. He is always braying at the five mini ponies standing next to the giant draft horse, Kate, asking them to slow down. Jack is a little slower than the rest, so his braying is a demand that they wait for him.

It's funny looking at a 2,000-pound horse next to a miniature pony weighing less than 200 pounds. Or a mini donkey that has had a stroke and one eye droops. His braying is a little off as well from the stroke. This is not expected in a small rural area 30 miles south of Atlanta. You would expect the occasional horse or assorted cows, but not camels or a water buffalo.

This strange sight only continues when I drive to the little town of Grantville. No grocery stores, too small, but there is a main street that is famous. It can be found in Season Three of the Walking Dead, in all of its glory, or the newest version of Dumb and Dumber 2. Recently, the entire downtown was auctioned off on eBay. No, you cannot make this stuff up.

I dodge flesh-eating zombies in downtown Grantville and the roadblocks that go up as they film. My husband works at the rock quarries where the invasions are going on *again* this year. They are continually filming the upcoming season. Yes, zombies and dynamite are the agenda of my husband's day. Arriving home, three camels, a water buffalo, and a donkey with a stroke greet my husband, and of course me, a wife with an incurable, rare cancer.

So how does this strange arrangement of animals from around the world and the Hollywood invasion of our little town, help explain my Medullary journey? Well, it's a story that is very true and very strange. The odds of taking a Sunday drive and seeing camels in someone's pasture with a water buffalo or a donkey that has had a stroke are greater than the odds of meeting a Medullary Thyroid Cancer patient in your entire life time. The odds of Hollywood wanting to use your little town to film zombies or Dumb and Dumber 2 are greater than your doctor diagnosing or treating a Medullary Thyroid Cancer patient.

Medullary is as rare as camels in Georgia.

Ever tried to get a large animal veterinarian to do a wellness check for a camel? I can tell you, they first run to a book, look up what they can on the Internet, and then tell you over and over again, "I've never done this before." Exactly the answers we medullary patients get from a primary care physician any time we go in for a wellness check.

Before 2009, you could not have told me that I would need a suitcase, a plane ticket, and comfortable shoes just to obtain blood work and a check-up on an incurable cancer. True life is stranger than fiction.

In Atlanta, thirty miles north of home, there's a hospital that can deal with the dreaded Ebola virus. Emory University and the CDC, side by side. But they can't deal with my Medullary and the results of massive neck surgeries. Medullary is very rare, but losing the thyroid and then the parathyroids as well is much more rare.

My journey began, as with most of us, with a simple yearly physical in 2009. Like most Meddies (that's what we call ourselves), we appear totally healthy. No labs or thyroid issues, nothing that would say, "You have Stage IV cancer." We all seem to be healthier than most, and all of us are very active people.

But I had a nagging pain in my right chest. I had unexplained diarrhea (a Meddie shared experience and the "butt" of most Meddie jokes), and hot flashes. The hot flashes were being blamed on my age. No labs, no questioning because I was so very healthy. As most of us would, I pressed the doctor about the nagging pain in the chest. "Well, we can do a chest x ray," was the simple answer.

A few days went by and I got a call. "Well, we see a golf ball in the right chest. Maybe you should see a pulmonologist." I called and it would be two months to see the pulmonologist. So I called a local general surgeon I knew.

I got the x-rays and as he walked in I proudly held them up for him. "Carol, didn't the doctor touch your neck?"

"It's in my chest and I want a piece of this to check it out," I proclaimed. The surgeon had not come through the door yet.

"No, did the other doctor do a *full* physical?"

"Yes," I proclaimed, "And right where the right chest hurts she says there's a golf ball and I want a piece of it," and I proudly held up the x-ray again.

"No." he yelled. "I'm asking about the neck. I can see the area from across the room and I haven't touched you yet."

"This is in the chest," I stated and again held up the x-ray.

"Shut up, Carol, and lie down. Whatever is in the chest came from the throat, and I can see that from across the room. You do know I don't do the chest, right?"

I will never forget that exchange. I was so shocked. I immediately shut up and lay down.

Within 48 hours, I'd had multiple labs, a full PET and CT scans with a plan to come back to his office for a biopsy. Best laid plans of mice and men, right?

Back to the general surgeon. The news was very strange. "Carol, I can't do a biopsy. I can't find a spot to put the needle. We can't see anything anywhere."

"Well, that's good news, right?" I asked.

"No, let me explain," was the answer.

The entire neck and all vital structures including veins, trachea, thyroid, right and left were encased in something that extended in one big lump into the chest. He could not find one spot to place a needle and not hit an artery that he could see, even with an ultrasound. "I want to take you into surgery to go way behind the left ear and try to cut a piece of this. If you bleed out, I'm not sure how to deal with this since everything is surrounding arteries."

He got a small piece in the hospital, of 1.5 centimeters. That was the small piece. He was afraid to go deeper or get the rest, and after surgery he told me they couldn't have stopped the bleeding in that artery if it broke. He also told me that surgery to remove this was not possible.

Now that did not seem right. It seemed strange. I have something that can't be removed? Let's find out what it is first, right?

Within one week the results came back. As I walked into the office with my sister, husband, daughter and son, I could see this surgeon's face turn white. He handed me what he could find from a medical journal. *Two* sentences.

In 30 years of practice, this general surgeon in a small rural town told me he had seen only one other medullary patient in his entire career. I asked what had happened to the patient. He told me the patient lived about 18 months.

He again told me that surgery was not an option. So after arguing the point with him, that *he* was not a chest surgeon, I went to Emory. I got him to call ahead and help expedite the appointments.

Emory wanted two months to order operating room equipment.

What is this two months thing? They wanted to do a *team* surgery with six surgeons. The neck, under collarbones and the chest would be done at the same time. Emory stated they had never done this type of big surgery, but they could try.

I asked simply, "Who has the equipment for this type of surgery?"

And that's where my entire life became even stranger. The answer was not in the state of Georgia, but only at large Centers of Cancer Excellence in much larger cities than Atlanta. The list included Mayo, Johns Hopkins, Sloane Kettering or MD Anderson. I called them all. MD Anderson did more Medullary patients than anyone.

At this point in my life, I had wanted to travel with my husband. My kids were over the age of 18, in college, and I wanted to have fun with the man who had become Dad. Be careful what you ask for. Off to Houston and major surgeries in 2009, and the trips will be made there for the rest of my life. The other major hospital I see every month is the National Institute of Health for a Clinical Trial. Traveling is a constant routine for all Medullary patients.

Besides constant travel, the Medullary patient also ends up with many blessings and losses that most cancer patients don't usually deal with. The biggest issue is the phrase "You don't look sick." Or "I had a friend who went through chemo or radiation and is just fine."

Then there are always the problems of talking with family. "You had a surgery and they got it all? ... So what's left can be gotten with chemo or radiation? ... I heard of this wonder food that will cure that ... You mean you must grow the tumor big enough to have another surgery? ... Why are you always traveling? ... Are you sure you still have cancer?"

Rare means you lose friends, and many times family members stop waiting for something to happen. Since there is no chemotherapy, no radiation, and only surgery, waiting until it is a matter of no choice before you have the next surgery to avoid scar tissue and complications makes most family members question what is going on.

Now, before I end my story, let me tell you how we ended up with something as rare as camels, a water buffalo, a donkey that has had a stroke, and five mini ponies?

Truly, when I met my husband Joseph, 33 years ago, I had no idea of the significance of his initials, and this has been the subject of many heated debates down the years.

They are J. H. C. Jr., so when I'm upset with him the swearing, "Okay, Jesus H. Christ Jr., have it your way!" can be heard loudly. Well, one day he told a lie to a neighbor just to get her dander up. He proclaimed that we were getting camels to be a pasture mate for Kate, the draft horse. Within three days God heard this lie and decided that J. H. C. Jr. needed to learn a lesson. A close friend called and was in need of help with an entire petting zoo that had been abandoned. From J.H.C. Jr.'s lips to God's ear, I'm blessed by my very rare life.

Circles

By Tamy Moretz

Life is full of circles. And what we decide to include in these circles makes our lives. Some circles are big, some are small, some change daily and some stay the same. But we all have circles.

Our families create one circle. The family is started with those who raise us and we are raised with, and the extended circles go out from there. As we grow, our family changes; we welcome new members as they are born or brought into our family. People pass away or walk out of our lives, and some families are created from circumstances. Our extended circles would include our work place, church, friends and health professionals such as doctors, preachers and sages.

These circles overlap and are ever changing.

A very wonderful circle in which I'm included is my meddie family! This circle of people has been a steadfast group, more than willing to do meet-ups, share experiences, celebrate for good results and mourn as a family when we lose a member. This has been an instrumental group in my journey. Without the knowledge of these people I would be lost in the dark and thinking I am cured because of a doctor's misinformation.

When you are dealing with a rare form of anything, knowledge is your major stabilizing point. Finding the correct people who know where and when to point you can be difficult, especially when dealing with doctors. I've been through five endocrinologists in three and a half years and only found one with any knowledge, Dr. Sherman. To say the least, I can tell you who *not* to go to in Nebraska.

The circle of doctors you choose to work with is an imperative part of your treatment plan. With endocrinologists, oncologists, radiologists, surgeons and more, the ability of these people to work together and with you, the patient is so important! If you can't work together to create a plan for treatment, or there is a lack of trust, then the circle will not be true.

The circle of friends is also challenging. When someone is diagnosed with cancer, they go through a litmus test with their friends. At this time people will find out who are the ones who'll stay and help and support, and who will walk out. This can be very daunting for the patient, as they believed that a person was there for them no matter what, and to watch them walk away is hard. To also have people jump on board to get the accolades for helping but not really investing is just wrong.

The best circle to find is the one where friends are willing to stay and help support you during your time. Some friends shy away, afraid of what to say or do. But the best thing is just to be there. You don't have to be cheerful at all times, or think you need to be Betty Bright. Be there to listen, to take out as a regular day. No cancer patient wants to be treated like they have the plague.

Needless to say, life is a circle from birth to death. Marriage rings are to show that it's an undying love, and then the friends each of us surrounds ourselves with create our CIRCLES.

Inner Voice

By Joyce Johnson

I used to enjoy talking
It was part of my soul
It was better than walking
It was the way that I rolled

But those days are gone
They are now in my past
Syllables, words and yes even song
Once taken for granted, they didn't last

Wanting to communicate, and to seek
Truth and information we long to share
Front and center is our beak
This is how we humans show that we care

Sad and lost, I felt for a time
Feeling the ravage of cancer
Forced into being an unpaid mime
Is akin to being a naked dancer

For the entire world to see, not hear
Struggling to make my thoughts known
Looking and searching; far and near
For another ability that I could hone

To cut to the chase
I'll tell you what this rhyme is about
Without further adieu and with much haste
I can no longer whisper, talk or shout

I have a nonverbal voice much wiser and older
And it no longer comes from my mouth
It's stronger, brighter and even bolder
Anatomically, it resides in a spot more south

It has more fully dawned on me
The importance of what's in our heart
Life is more than what we touch, taste and see
It's the meaning of our being that's the superior part

This nonverbal voice has taught me much more
My value is based not on what I say
My value is much deeper, rooted in my core
And life is grand, come what may

Even though cancer has pillaged and taken
This new normal is not all bad
I refuse to be ignored or forsaken
My life is the opposite of weakened or sad.

Em Tough, Fight Like A Girl

By Hope Koehler

We haven't been on our journey long, but it's definitely one I wish for no one. We're a typical Midwestern family of four, consisting of Dad, Rich, Mom, Hope, and two girls, Kayla, 17, Emily, 11. We live in a rural community and our girls go to the same school from which both Rich and I graduated. Life has been good! We are blessed with great family and friends. We have worked hard for everything we have, and overall are very content with our lives. We'd never have anticipated hearing the words that our daughter, Emily, had cancer, and then dealing with the rarity of Medullary Thyroid Carcinoma (MTC). Why do I tell you this? Because cancer does not discriminate against anyone! Young, old, of different skin color, poor or rich, it happens.

Emily's journey started with neck swelling, headaches and weight loss. In early 2014 Emily had the typical common cold, with swollen lymph nodes. Unfortunately, the swelling never went down, and symptoms became worse. The headaches were happening daily and the neck movement was very restricted. I requested to see an ENT (Ear Nose and Throat doctor). My husband, Rich, brought Emily to the ENT, who scheduled an MRI of her neck the following week. Unfortunately, the doctor could not determine what was in her neck and referred us to Children's Hospital in Madison.

We met with a doctor on November 10 at University of Wisconsin (UW) Health Children's Hospital. After looking at the MRI he declared in his best professional doctor's voice, "Emily you have a blob in your neck!" The only way to determine what was wrong with Emily was to schedule a surgery to look at her neck. We had surgery scheduled for November 13.

Emily is no stranger to surgeries or the Children's Hospital, as in the past she had had both her knees operated on there. She was brave, as always, and wasn't really that nervous. Honestly, I don't think Rich and I were, either, as she had always been a healthy girl except for her knees. She went in to surgery and Rich and I went back to the pre-op room. An hour or so passed and the doctor returned to the room with an update.

The update no parent wants to hear. During the surgery he was able to biopsy two lymph nodes. The pathologist immediately determined they were malignant. Devastating! Tears, shock and disbelief overwhelmed us, and the doctor left so we could regain our composure before seeing Emily in recovery.

We were admitted to the Oncology floor. I was fortunate in that an RN whom I had previously worked with had moved to Madison and worked on that floor. She was a lifesaver and was able to reassure us that they would get Emily the best treatment. We met with Emily's oncologist. Oncologist. What a strange word for us to say about our 11-year-old.

More tests were needed to determine what type of cancer she had. I really can't remember much except that Emily was tired, cranky and wanted to go home. The oncologist met with me in the morning and determined it was a type of thyroid cancer, but needed a few more tests. Oblivious, I thought, "Okay, let's remove the thyroid. Yes, she'll need to be on medication the rest of her life, but we can handle this."

WRONG! CT scan was performed and an MRI was scheduled. That night we were unable to get the MRI, as the hospital had many other cases. The oncologist told us Emily had MTC, a rare cancer that could be very hard to detect. That was all I really knew or heard. We were sent home that night and an MRI was scheduled for another day.

Another trip to Madison! MRI was done November 18 and we met with the oncologist and surgeon, who gave us more heart-wrenching news. The cancer had metastasized, which meant it had spread. They found spots on her liver and noticed some abnormalities in her spine. The neck mass was wrapped around her carotid artery, and if surgery were performed it would be very complicated. Her blood levels were high at CEA 17.8 and calcitonin more than 28,000. So many people were in the room, and everyone was so quiet. Rich and I just cried.

Believe me, my head was down and I only heard half of what they said. Before a treatment plan of any source could be made we needed a bone scan. We had been praying so hard for it to come back negative.

The scan was performed on November 20 and we were to meet with the oncologist on November 26. The results showed several different areas of concern, and there were spots on the liver.

Because of the rarity of this cancer, our oncologist had contacted specialists around the world to look at Emily's case. She had reached out to MD Anderson Hospital in Houston, Texas, which had many providers with knowledge of MTC. I also learned about this Facebook support group for MTC, my new family of "Meddies."

The oncologist told us about an oral pill, approved for adults that slowed down this cancer, but it had not been approved for Pediatrics. She was working on getting Emily approved through a hospital in Chicago.

While all this was going on we had great support from family, friends and community. The teachers and staff at our daughter's school were amazing, and they showed so much support, compassion and loyalty to our family. We are very blessed to have them all in our lives.

On December first I received great news from our insurance company. They had approved Emily to see the MTC Specialist at MD Anderson. One more trip to Madison to talk with doctors and the social worker on how our family was coping. With our heads just above water it seemed we heard more and more bad news about this cancer. We knew only one case in one million kids who had this. Emily had a better chance winning the lottery.

We flew to Texas on December 7. Rich wasn't able to make this trip, but we are very lucky to have Aunt Julie come along for support. Emily did great for a first-time flyer. The airports were very quiet and we had no trouble at all. We were greeted by Jan, one of Julie's coworker's aunts, who was simply amazing.

Texas is not a bit like Wisconsin! There were a billion hospitals in one area. Emily and I weren't used to the big city. We stayed at the Rotary House, which is connected to MD Anderson. The hotel has 11 levels, and we were on the 10th. We got our new patient information, walked around in the hotel and had frozen yogurt, then went to see a movie. The pool and fitness center was open 24/7, and Emily loved the pool.

The next day we saw Dr. Waguespack, who was very nice and Emily liked him. It was another information overload, but Julie was along to transcribe. Emily was scheduled for blood work, an ultrasound, CT scans and MRIs. The next step was to talk with Dr. Clayman about surgery and see if this was the right path to take. Dr. Waguespack had only seen five kids with this cancer, and there was complexity in the way the tumor was growing in her neck.

We met with Dr. Clayman, who would be performing Emily's surgery. He said that even with this rare cancer, she had an even rarer case because it was not a typical MTC tumor in her neck. The mass had intertwined through veins, arteries and vocal chords. His statement was "This is very strange." I asked if he felt he could remove some of the tumor, and his statement was "I'm removing it all and I'm the only one in the world who can do this!" All I could think was thank God this is the answer we've been looking for. He told Emily not to worry, as he had been in this rodeo before.

We headed back to Wisconsin to enjoy our Christmas before surgery in January.

During the week we were home, it was a roller coaster filled with tears, sadness, fear, laughter, and joy. We knew we had a difficult road ahead of us but we were going to get through this. Reading the doctors' reports and the words "Stage 4 cancer" was so frightening. There were days when I didn't even want to wake up and have to deal with this, and then the days when I was up all night with a wandering mind and a box of Kleenex. People stopped in and asked questions, which was exhausting as we tried to explain. Then there were those who said, "Oh, this person had thyroid cancer and they just took out the thyroid and they were fine." HA HA! If I had a dollar for every time I'd heard that in the last six months, I'd be rich.

Overall, Emily was very tired, whether it was from the cancer or the emotions she was going through, it was very difficult seeing her like this, especially being a parent who couldn't fix her own child. According to her doctors she needed to gain weight. Her appetite had been fairly good and she understood that she needed to eat to keep up her strength. She was so tired she missed school, and she simply didn't feel like doing much.

Emily and I flew back to MD Anderson on January 9 for more tests and a pre-op visit with Dr. Waguespack, Dr. Clayman, and Dr. Yu. We were blessed to meet a wonderful "meddie" family whom we prayed with and had a wonderful talk with over lunch. Emily said he reminded her of Grandpa.

Rich and Kayla flew in on January 12 so they could be here for Emily's surgery. This was Kayla's first time flying and it was not something she enjoyed.

Surgery was scheduled for January 15. The plastic surgeon would be removing a section in her upper thigh to knee area, depending on how much he needed to reconstruct the neck. The leg part took about an hour, and then reconstruction of the neck would take about three hours, as the surgeon would need to attach veins and arteries under a microscope. The procedure is called a "flap." The thoracic surgeon would also be taking a section from an artery in her leg and using it to repair her carotid artery, if needed. There are four main arteries in the neck, so one can be shut down for a bit to be replaced, and if her artery didn't work they would put in an artificial one. Amazing what these talented doctors can do! Emily would be taken to ICU after surgery, as they didn't want her to wake up right away after such a complicated procedure.

Surgery time arrived. We were to check in at 5:30a.m. The line for checking in was so long I couldn't believe all these people needed surgery. The wait to be called back was about an hour, and then everything happened so fast. Many doctors and nurses went in and out of the room. An IV was started, gown and cap were put on and she was ready. Then the separation anxiety began. She was scared, and tears flowed, and she didn't want to go through this. They gave her some anti-anxiety medications and her favorite stuffed animal, Wolfie. We kissed her good-bye and then the doors were shut as she was rolled into the procedure area. Of course, the first place my mind went to was, "Is this going to be the last time we see her? Will she feel pain? Was this the right thing to do?" So many questions.

Surgery began at 7:14am. They started incisions at 8:19. They estimated eight hours from 8:19a.m. We were told that we would receive regular updates. The first would be around 10:00a.m. Emily was in stable condition. The waiting was unbearable. Finally, Kayla came and we decided we should get something to eat.

Second Update was at 2:44p.m. Amazingly, Dr. Clayman was able to remove the entire tumor in the neck on both sides. The left side was getting as bad as the right. He removed all lymph nodes on both sides, the thyroid, and the right vocal cord. He basically cleaned out her whole neck. He was able to save her carotid, so hadn't needed the thoracic surgeon. Dr. Clayman said it could not have gone better. The plastic surgeon was putting in the flap, so it would be a few hours yet.

Third Update. Still stable, and the plastic surgeon was still working on the flap. She had not needed a blood transfusion up to that point, so still good news.

Fourth Update at 4:53p.m. Plastic surgeon was done. They had taken the right upper muscle out of her leg and wrapped it around the neck from the left side over the windpipe to the right side. They'd found tumors around the trachea, and removed them. Now hopefully the tissues would all take. Emily was getting cleaned up and then they'd take her to ICU.

We waited and waited for what seemed like hours to see which room they were taking her to. Doctors were leaving, and the waiting room—which had once been so full—had only a few people left. I asked volunteers for help, and they called the nurse, who told us it would be hours yet, as the plastic surgeon was still working on her. WHAT?! I'd talked to the surgeon an hour ago and he was done. What was she talking about?

After a few phone calls she was able to tell us Emily was in ICU and we needed to go there. Going into ICU was a nightmare. Emily was awake and crying, and she was trying to scream. The nurse looked at us and said, "About time you get here"!

They had to be kidding me. I was pissed and told her we'd been in the waiting room all this time and they'd told us Emily was still in surgery. We left this ugly situation and comforted Emily as much as we could.

The nights were long and the nurses were horrible. Emily wasn't able to get out of bed because she was so medicated and in pain, and every time she needed to use the bathroom we needed to call for help. That was like asking them to give up their right arm. Medication wasn't working and I requested that she be switched to something else. Finally, after a few hours we had a nurse change and this nurse listened to us. Things were looking up. However, in the following nights, we still had the night nurse we all dreaded. She was a traveling nurse and had never worked in a Pediatric ICU setting. She would not keep the flap area moist, even after my request and the doctors insisting it needed to be done. The worst night was when she got Emily out of bed and onto the commode. Then she walked away, leaving Emily naked. She said, "I'm going to get supplies to wash her up."

Seriously? Lady, have you ever heard of a fall risk?! By the time she'd come back Emily was in pain and wanted to go back to bed. The nurse was so mad at her she whipped off her gloves and walked out of the room. I was so pissed I didn't know what to do. I got Emily back into a gown and helped her into bed. She finally rested that night.

Other nights were worse. She'd scream at us to leave and go back to Wisconsin. All three of us left the room crying and I watched her fragile body shake through the observation window. I stayed in the ICU for six days while Rich and Kayla went back to the hotel. I was so afraid to leave Emily with these nurses! I did file a complaint and was told someone would contact me. Almost four months later, still nothing. Dr. Waguespack and his nurse were so sorry to hear about our experience, as they said they'd never had a patient who'd needed to go into ICU after a surgery like this.

Four days after surgery things were finally looking brighter. Emily was eating and working on physical therapy. Her spirit had lifted and I think she knew she had to gain strength so we could go back home.

In the meantime, it was time for Dad and Kayla to go back home. That was a hard day. I didn't want them to leave and I didn't know how I was going to take care of her by myself. Fortunately, I had Jan close by, who came and visited and called and texted daily. An angel in disguise. The nights were lonely without having Rich to talk to and then hearing all the fun stuff they were doing at home. I was jealous, I know, but how come I had to be the one to do this?

Six days after being admitted to ICU we were able to go back to the Rotary House. Emily was still weak, but I was able to get her around in a wheelchair, and we toured the hospital. We found lots of interesting places, like Kim's place, a hangout for teenagers. We also had fun while we were there we spent a whole day at the Houston Zoo, from opening to close. We ate with the giraffes and had some great laughs. We also had some low moments when people stared and asked what happened to her. Emily's standard reply was, "I got my head chopped off and sewed back on." Oh, boy, did that scare them away! The Rotary House was great and had lots of free entertainment to enjoy. We even met a 20-year-old who had cancer and talked to Emily about how brave she was. We met another "meddie," and she gave Emily a beautiful scarf to wear. It was great, the support we received.

There are days that are better than others, and it's very hard not to think about what's going to happen in our future. It's amazing how things have changed in such a short time. You really learn a lot about people when you have to go through an event like this. Some people feel it's better to leave you alone and not talk about what you're going through. Unfortunately, that makes it feel like they don't care. I've seen people at the store who've said, "I was hoping not to run into you because I don't know what to say."

How brutal. Others just don't understand, and say she looks fine.

I've found it easier to avoid these people and will even drive out of my way to go to another grocery store. It was initially overwhelming, with everyone wanting to see Emily and us, and then it was like everyone dropped off the face of earth. I think you find out who your real friends are in a situation like this.

Since surgery, Emily has had many ER visits. Her calcium has been very low and her thyroid has fluctuated. It's a balancing act, and I know it'll take time for her body to adjust. The worst has been the tingling sensation she gets over her entire body. Hopefully, we'll get answers to all this soon.

As I write this, Rich, Kayla and I had our genetic testing. Thank God Rich and Kayla are negative, but I'm positive for the RET mutation. Again, WHY? To find out I have the same RET mutation as Emily and that it's genetic is very hard to deal with. Knowing I've passed this terrible disease to her. Listening to doctors tell me I need to have surgery and wondering how I can be gone and not be there for my family is heartbreaking. To hear people say, "If you need anything, let me know" is the worst. We need lots of things, but really I don't have the time to tell you what we need. Sometimes the little gestures without us asking are the greatest things. The best laugh I got was when someone asked, "This makes no sense you have this. Is it contagious, do you think it's in the water?" No, it's hereditary!

I am so thankful that we have an amazing school system with wonderful teachers and staff who are there for Emily and Kayla every day. It actually gives me peace when Emily is at school because I know she's keeping herself occupied, and she has many watching over her.

I have to give Rich much credit, as I know this is so hard on him and he's handling everything so well. We have many tearful nights. Days when we don't want to look at each other and days that are filled with much happiness.

Our family cannot express our thanks for what everyone is doing for us with cards, gifts, donations and prayers. It's truly amazing!! As Dr. Waguespack said, as of 2014, there's no cure for this cancer, but with all the research they're doing we're very hopeful that some light can be given to all cancer patients. We have one tough young lady here, and with everyone's support I know Emily can fight and stay strong!!

I'm very thankful to have found the "Meddie" group. They definitely are family, and I can reach out to them any time I need to, day or night. My prayers to all of them and their families, because this is such a long road to walk.

As I finish writing this we'll leaving for MD Anderson for a recheck. Our journey has just begun.

POEM:

Our story is us.
Our story is real.
But now how do we deal?
Another visit or retreat.
We are done! We are beat!
We know we are tough,
But, hey, we've had enough.
Is this a bad dream?
Then why do I hear myself scream?
We can't answer the reasons why,
So more tears we will cry.
Another day it will be
We will fight this, just wait and see!

My MEN IIB Story

By Elizabeth Eastburn

From reading others' stories on Facebook, I consider myself very fortunate to have known about my diagnosis from the beginning of my memory. My father had MENIIB but wasn't diagnosed until his early teens, by his ophthalmologist actually. He died from complications of MTC when I was 8 years old, but my mother is a tumor registrar so she has researched this syndrome extensively and is a wealth of knowledge when I or my doctors have questions. With her cancer knowledge and background, she understands more about my syndrome than I ever will. I also had the help of my oncologist, who my mother knew professionally for years. My mother didn't like any endocrinologists around so I've seen this oncologist for as long as I can remember.

From as far back as I can remember, I was tested several times a year for my syndrome. These blood and urine tests were an inconvenience but part of my life. I was born with club feet, which isn't a diagnosed symptom of this disorder, but several doctors believe it is part of the syndrome. My right foot was operated on several times but my left foot was fixed with foot braces. Today, my right foot is a size 6 and my left foot is a size 8. Shoe shopping is the bane of my existence. My thyroid was removed when I was 4 years old. There was a little cancer in it and since it was all removed, I never had to endure chemo or radiation. I also got to keep my lymph nodes as they were free of cancer. In December 2001, I had symptoms of my first pheochromocytoma on my right adrenal gland. I was in college and would get a fast heartbeat while in class and after a couple days of this, I told my mother who immediately scheduled me for a CT scan and MRI, which revealed the tumor. My right adrenal gland was removed in Dec. 2001 and I healed nicely, though I was told to watch for other symptoms and would do other testing to watch my remaining adrenal gland since that's the most likely place a second tumor would locate itself. In early 2010, after my yearly testing, I got home and was called by my doctor saying they saw something on my adrenal and I would need further testing. Sure enough, a second pheo was found, though I had no symptoms this time. Bad timing for me as my fiancé and I were planning our wedding for April and my sister's wedding was planned for May that year. Since I had no symptoms and having both adrenals removed would bring about changes in my life that could affect both weddings, we decided to wait until after both weddings to have it removed.

In early July 2010, my second adrenal was removed, this time laparoscopically. Turns out, your adrenals do more for your body than you can ever imagine. I was discharged from the ICU but didn't listen to doctors' orders to literally do *nothing* but rest, and after a couple times of going up and down stairs to get things for myself and doing a couple loads of dishes, I was in the hospital for exhaustion. After being told to *really* not do anything but rest, I listened. So my 6 weeks off work were spent learning how much energy it takes to do everyday things and working out how much of the steroids I was now prescribed to take to get through the day.

I have had years to figure out how to live with no adrenal glands now and I know what my body is capable of fighting off and when I will need more steroids, but it's still hard at times to accept that I can't heal or fight off things like I used to do easily. I work in a preschool, a petri dish of germs, but I keep myself healthy for the most part. I get the occasional sinus infection, asthma attack, pink eye, etc. but when I have more than one infection in me, that's when I can get into trouble and need medical help to fight them off. I can feel myself drained of energy depending on how much energy I have expended with activities, and I know when to slow it down and rest, which is hard at times. One major change since having my adrenals removed is my body temperature. Pre-surgeries, when I had at least one adrenal, I was always cold. I would wear jackets with everything; get cold feet and hands through all the seasons. After taking out the second adrenal gland, I rarely get cold. In fact, I go around with no coat for most of the year and get hot doing normal things through the day. I still bring a jacket with me sometimes just in case I go into an unusually cold place, but rarely do I need to wear them.

I look forward to learning from others who might be like me as I have never met another person with my syndrome.

Medullary Thyroid Cancer: Story Of Miracles

By Virginia Skilton

In the late summer of 2009 I decided I was tired of the upper back and neck pain I'd been having for months. My general practitioner referred me to an orthopedic spine doctor, Dr. E. at the Orthopedic Clinic. He ordered physical therapy and massage to help with the back and neck spasms, and then ordered an MRI. When I went back to see him, he said many people would love to have my spine. But while there were no problems with my spine, he did see a nodule on my thyroid and suggested I have it checked. He didn't push the issue, just left it up to me to decide.

Miracle number one.

I knew of our local general surgeon in the neighboring town and made an appointment to see what he had to say about the thyroid nodule. He checked the CD of my MRI and felt my neck. He decided to do a fine needle aspiration (FNA) to see if there were any cancer cells in the nodule on the left side of the thyroid gland. He injected some lidocaine in the front of my neck and proceeded to do four or five biopsies. Even with the lidocaine the procedure was very painful.

After a week of waiting he called me in to discuss the test results. I felt scared and was afraid of bad news. However, I was surprised when he said there wasn't any cancer evident within the nodule. He said we could leave it and watch it over time, or we could take it out. I heard a voice in my head say loud and clear: "Take it out!" In fact, it was so loud and clear I actually laughed about it later. When I told the doctor to take it out he had a surgical appointment for me the very next week.

Miracle number two.

I had my total thyroidectomy (TT) on November 4, 2009, at the local county hospital in our small city. During the surgery, Dr. S. decided to biopsy the right side of my thyroid. The preliminary results showed Hurthle cells. Dr. S. decided to remove the complete thyroid gland and some lymph nodes around it. He also removed one parathyroid gland, but left the other three in place.

It was a big surprise to my family that I had cancer and that it had spread, as half of the lymph nodes they removed also had cancer. My family had been in the waiting room to see the doctor after surgery. I was also surprised, but not as much as my family, as I felt that it was my destiny to have it. Anyway, it was my cross to bear and I was going to bear it the best I could. Chin up and carry on, and all that stuff.

My stay in the hospital was just overnight, and I went home the next day with a drain and a dressing on my neck. I had staples in my incision and had to wear a bandage for nearly a week, after which I would go back and have the staples removed. I also had a damaged vocal cord and couldn't speak above a whisper, although the doctor said it would get better over time. My husband joked to our family that he'd paid extra to have it done so I couldn't yell at him! It was his way of deflecting the seriousness of my diagnosis, as he was afraid for what was ahead.

A week later I returned to have my staples removed. We carried on a little bit of a conversation, and after the staples were removed and the bandage replaced, the surgeon asked my husband and me to come into his office. He actually had tears in his eyes when he started to tell us about the pathology report, which showed medullary thyroid cancer (MTC) instead of the Hurthle cells found during surgery. It was extremely serious, and I would need more surgeries that would be severely disfiguring and disabling. I might need a tracheotomy and feeding tube. Moreover, my future prognosis was not good, as this was a very aggressive cancer.

I tried to keep the positive attitude I'd been working on since my cancer diagnosis, but it was so difficult. Even though he was trying to not let me see how afraid he was, I could still see the shock on my husband's face. We left the doctor's office and went to my son's house, as he was home from working the night shift. When we told him, he was stoic, but he hugged me so long and hard, I knew he was also afraid of what was in my future.

We told our other son later, as he was at work at the time. Our daughter had to be told in a phone call, and I knew how hard it was for her to hear this about me. It made things even harder, as we lived so far from each other.

My surgeon suggested I go to a large teaching hospital about an hour from us, as they would have more experience with MTC and would have genetic doctors who could explain it further and provide the necessary testing to determine if it was the genetic or sporadic kind of medullary. His office staff helped set up an appointment for me and faxed my medical information to them.

I had to get my pathology slides sent to the larger hospital and had to go to the pathology lab at our county hospital to request that they be sent out. One of the pathologists heard me making the request and came over to talk with me. He was the pathologist who had dissected my tumor and found the medullary. He told me he had seen this kind of cancer before, as he used to work at the large teaching hospital where I was being referred. There had never been a case of MTC diagnosed at our local hospital.

Miracle number three.

Telling the rest of my family was fairly straightforward. There is no beating around the bush when it's cancer and when there's a possibility it's genetic and they could have it, too. So the wheels started turning.

I saw the genetic counselor and genetic doctor within a few weeks. After blood draws to check for the genetic marker, I had to wait again. In the meantime I had my first visit with an endocrinologist, but I didn't care for her flippant attitude. She brushed me off by telling me this cancer was not a big deal and that I was fine. I didn't feel fine at that point. I was afraid and didn't know what was going to be in my future.

I also had an appointment with the endocrine surgeon. I liked him. He did an ultrasound and saw some suspicious nodes in the left side of my neck, so he followed up with fine needle aspirations, with no medication to numb my neck. This made me very uncomfortable. I wanted to cry after that, but I just rode home with an ice pack on my neck and held all the emotion inside.

After a week of waiting for the lab results from the biopsies, I discovered they were positive for cancer, which meant they needed to come out. A surgery was scheduled for January 11, 2010, for a modified radical left neck dissection. I was so afraid of what my future would hold that I don't think I even breathed for weeks on end. I just held my breath and waited for the other shoe to drop. I had a constant prayer going round and round in my head to help me be strong and not be a burden to my husband and family.

I arrived very early at the clinic for my surgery. The incision went from just right of the end of the TT incision to below my ear on the left neck. I was out of surgery by 10:30 a.m. The surgeon said everything went well and there were no issues. But as a result I had numbness on the left side of my face, ear, neck, and into my shoulder. I also had limited left arm movement.

I was sent home the day after my surgery on January 12, 2010. I went back for drain removal a couple of days later. I had a drain from the incision, which was closed with stitches inside and glue outside.

It looked much better than the incision from my first surgery. I would measure the fluid from the drain bulb daily and record the amount. I didn't like the drain bulb dangling so I pinned it with a safety pin to my shirt. There were so many new things to get used to with these surgeries. When the fluid began to decrease they took out the drain. I did not feel well most of the time and guessed this would be my new normal

On January 28 I had a PET scan, a CT scan of head and neck, and a liver scan. Thankfully, all the results were normal, but I did have some spots in my lungs. The doctors didn't think it was cancer, but would monitor them just to be sure. I also had a consultation with the genetic counselor and genetic doctor. They were very helpful and gave us a great deal of printed information to read about medullary and familial genetic markers. I had a blood draw that checked the genetic marker for Multiple Endocrine Neoplasia type 2 (MEN2a). This was very frightening to me because if I had a genetic marker, then the rest of my family would have to be tested. A large group of family members could potentially be affected.

On February 15, I called the genetic counselor, but there were as yet no test results. On February 16 I had a bone scan at our local hospital. This required an injection at 9 a.m. and then a scan at noon. The scan took about 40 minutes and the technician repeated some areas just to be thorough. I wondered if there was a problem. (My mind seemed to go to the worst-case scenario lately.)

We met with the genetic counselor on March 11. The testing showed a RET proto-oncogene mutation, exon 15 S891A DNA change 2671T-G (TCG>GCG) RET, low risk for aggression. This was MEN2a. The bottom line was that my immediate family would have to be tested for this marker. My three brothers and nephew, along with my children and our grandchildren if their parents were positive. Then, if any of them had the marker their children would have to be tested, and so on down the lines of generations. My counselor gave us a huge quantity of information and letters to share my diagnosis information with my family members.

On March 13 my husband and I had a get-together at our home

for my brothers, nephew and our sons to explain to them what was happening to me and ask them to please consider testing to see if they were positive for MEN2a. We didn't have any family history of thyroid cancer or the other health issues that can be associated with MEN2a, so I was declared the "de novo case," which means the first to be diagnosed. If we'd been aware of the genetic defect earlier, I wouldn't have been a Stage 3 at diagnosis. Everyone was willing to go to the clinic for a counseling session and then have their blood tested to check for the genetic marker.

Thankfully, I held it together emotionally, even though all I wanted to do was break down and cry. This would be a terrible burden on my extended family if anyone had the gene. I prayed no one else would have it.

I prepared a nice dinner for everyone. Food seems to help everyone get through some of the rough spots and makes them seem not so bad. I made BBQ pulled pork, cheesy potatoes, cole slaw and relish tray, chips, dip, pretzels and nacho chips. My nephew's wife and my daughter-in-law brought delicious desserts. Our meeting went well. We enjoyed our time together despite the reason for the meeting. I felt so much support for everything my husband and I were dealing with.

On March 25 my sons, three brothers and nephew had their appointments to visit the genetic counselor and get answers to questions regarding the impact this could have on their families. They each decided to have the testing to check them for the marker. If they tested positive it could affect many more of the family. My older brother even has great grandchildren. Several weeks went by. On April 7 they got their results.

Another miracle.

My brothers and nephew were all negative for the genetic marker. However, my sons were both positive, so their children needed to be tested. Our daughter also had the gene, which meant her children had to be tested. There was a 50/50 chance with each of my pregnancies to have the gene, and every one of mine got it! (I think we should have played the lottery with odds like this!)

Our eldest son's two boys were tested and they didn't have the gene. Our youngest son's two children both tested positive, and of our daughter's three children, the two youngest were positive. So out of our seven grandchildren, four were positive and three were negative for the genetic marker of MEN2a.

This summer will be a busy surgery time as each of our children has calcitonin (tumor marker) indicated in the testing. Our two sons who live locally are scheduled for June 7. We plan to be there, and then plan to watch the grandchildren while their fathers recuperate. Our daughter who lives in Illinois will have her surgery on June 24. We plan to travel there to be with her and the children during the surgery and beyond. It will be a 435-mile drive, but I'm willing to be with her and help out as much as I can. It's tough, though, because I still feel unwell so much of the time.

Our children all have MTC, and the youngest also has papillary cancer, plus he has cancer outside the thyroid and into his lymph nodes. Nine of fifteen nodes tested positive. He will have to have the radioactive iodine (RAI) treatment to kill the papillary cancer, and his thyroid stimulating hormone (TSH) will be suppressed to help combat the development of more papillary cancer.

When I had my first biopsy there were also papillary cells within the thyroid. I was not informed of this at the time, and only found out because my endocrine surgeon was keeping my TSH so suppressed and I asked why. I wondered if that was why I was feeling so poorly, but everyone passed it off, saying it was due to the challenging emotional year I'd been having. (What I was learning was that it paid to educate myself on these things.)

We went to Illinois on July 21 to be with our grandchildren, aged nine and eleven, for their thyroidectomy surgery. They did well during surgery, but our grandson had very low calcium, so they stayed over for two nights. We had one-on-one time with our eldest granddaughter while the younger ones were in the hospital and mom and dad were staying with them. I believe she felt guilty because she didn't have this issue to deal with like her siblings. Still, it's hard to know what others are thinking through any situation.

We stayed until the kids were out of the hospital. A few days later our granddaughter was already asking to ride her bike! The kids were such troupers through everything. It's so heartbreaking for me that they have to experience all the pain from the surgery and the testing while they are so young. They are very good about taking their daily medications. The best thing is that results from their pathology show that they are both free of MTC. Yay!!

Miracle number . . . ? I've lost count.

I have had such a pain in my heart this whole year for what I passed on to my precious family. All those years ago my husband and I were told we couldn't have children. So we decided to adopt, and had gone through all the interviewing, letters from friends and the doctor and meetings with a group of people who wanted to adopt. We had turned in our final paperwork and all we had to do was to wait for a baby.

A few weeks later I found out I was expecting. We were overjoyed. We canceled the adoption proceedings and awaited our baby. All I ever wanted was to be a mother, and my dreams and wishes were coming true. Little did I know at that time the heartache, pain and financial burden I would be giving to my precious children. I guess it's a great thing we don't have a crystal ball to foretell our future, or we may never do the things we do. I simply can't imagine life without my children.

On June 8, 2011, our next grandchild, nine-year-old daughter of our youngest son, had her surgery. My surgeon assisted her pediatric surgeon in performing a complete thyroidectomy and also removing a couple of lymph nodes. They found microscopic medullary cancer within the thyroid. Damn! The one thing I didn't want to have happen had happened. I was so heartbroken for her and her family. I was afraid for her future. She did well and stayed overnight. I'm so proud of my little warrior.

On July 6 I had an appointment with my surgeon and the ultrasound showed more lymph nodes that needed to be removed. My husband saw them quite clearly on the ultrasound screen and knew it was not good news without even being told. An ultrasound-guided fine needle aspiration was set up immediately. Once again I didn't get any numbing shot. The needles were very long as the nodes were deep. It hurt so badly as he probed the nodes. He even had to get a more powerful ultrasound to show the nodes clearly enough for the FNA. At one point he hit a nerve to my shoulder and arm and the pain was awful. He apologized, but the deed had been done. It hurt for hours afterward.

Two of the five biopsies were inconclusive, but the others were positive. Surgery was scheduled right away. Here we go again!

On August 1, 2011, my surgeon performed a selective neck dissection. We left home at 4:30 a.m. to get to the hospital early enough for all the set-up. The surgery took three and one-half hours and went well. I was released the next morning. Several days later the pathology came back indicating they had found cancer in four of the fourteen lymph nodes removed. So far about half of all the lymph nodes removed in my three surgeries had been positive for MTC.

In December our six-year-old grandson will have his surgery during Christmas break. He does really well and doesn't let much keep him down. He has a diagnosis of microscopic medullary within the thyroid, as did his nine-year-old sister. Their father, our youngest son, was the one who had both medullary and papillary. He had to undergo the RAI treatment only one time, and so far has not had to repeat it. I am thankful the doctors caught it when they did.

From this time forward I will be tested every six months. My family also has this time schedule for testing, and everyone has remained stable. I am so sorry for what my family has had to endure, and what they will always have to monitor. I do know I'm blessed in many ways by having children and grandchildren who don't blame me for what I passed on to them. It could have been much worse, and I'm grateful for that. Of course, my ultimate wish is that it had never happened, but if it was to happen, then I'm glad it happened when it did so my family could be spared a much worse prognosis. I've always been a positive person and counted my blessings daily long before this experience, challenge, war, or whatever you'd call it. I'm so thankful we're all doing fairly well and now can just keep on keeping on.

I hope the best for each of my meddie brothers and sisters. We're all family, and I appreciate each of you and the support you've given me during the past five years. We've had our share of miracles.

I wish some for you, too.

Support Is Crucial

By Vickie Baggett

I was the first in my family to be diagnosed with medullary thyroid cancer, along with a rare genetic mutation called multiple endocrine neoplasia, or MEN. Medullary thyroid cancer is one part of the MEN syndrome. The other parts are hyperparathyroidism and pheochromocytoma (tumor on your adrenal glands).

Getting diagnosed with MEN can be difficult at best. Once you're diagnosed, find a support group right away. They'll know who the experts are and where you should go to get the best treatment. During my 15 years I have learned to appreciate family, friends, and each other every day.

If I could impart one piece of wisdom, it would be that life is what happens in between the doctor's appointments. Don't live your life from test to test, or doctor's appointment to doctor's appointment. Make as many memories as possible with those you love.

There is a great support group and website for all thyroid cancers called ThyCa. The website is www.thyca.org. You can also find them on Facebook. Everyone there is very supportive.

The website and support group for MEN is called AMEND. The website is www.amendusa.org. They are also on Facebook and are very supportive and know what you're going through.

You are not alone in this! You might lose a friend or two along the way because they don't understand what you're going through. However, you'll find others going through the same thing you are, and may become fast friends.

Seek out help. Enjoy every day.

Cancer Changes The Meanings Of Four Words

By William Kenly
Author of The Dogs of Cancer, The Dogs of Divorce, and The Dogs of Luck

1. HOPE

Good topic.
Sorta like motherhood and apple pie.
Gotta have hope, don't we?
Parents name their children "Hope".
Churches promise that we will have it if we will just believe.
But what is it, really?

I started my relationship with "Hope" in 2001,
When my wife of 24 years served me with divorce papers.
I bled, but I survived.
But in its wake, it left a new horizon.
I was no longer looking for future fulfillment.
My horizon was measured in days or weeks,
But not much in years anymore.
I adopted a new mantra, "Keep Moving."
I understood a new truth:

"Yesterday and tomorrow are thieves that rob me of my todays."
I become more spiritual and less religious,
And so I was not inundated with promises of "Hope" as often,
Because I didn't go to church as often.

And I wrote a book about "Hope", *The Dogs of Divorce,* as therapy.

Seven years later, my relationship with "Hope" entered a new phase,
When I was diagnosed with a rare
And aggressive form of thyroid cancer.
One of cancer's benefits is that you find a new perspective on time.
My horizon shrank, again.
I concentrated very hard on enjoying today.
Every day I asked myself, and my new wife,
"What was the best thing that happened today?"
As my head was hitting the pillow each night,
I searched my memory for the "good" from today.
And I took that "good" to sleep with me.

And I wrote, *The Dogs of Cancer,* as therapy.

And so today, I don't care much for "Hope".
Did I have the best day today?
Tomorrow will be what it will be.
My "Hope" will not change that.
My prayers might, but that's a different topic.
In fact, "Hope" is rather false.
It's like "Tomorrow".
And we have already discussed how "Tomorrow" is a thief
That robs us of today.
Sorry. I don't want to take "Hope" away from anyone.
I would like to help them find "Today".
Enjoy "Today".

2. STRENGTH

Strange word,
Like big muscles,
Hard head,
Happy spirit,
Different after diagnosis than before.
Be strong, Bill.

Ability to proceed,
Ability to sustain,
Ability by oneself,
Ability to adapt,
Different levels of understanding.
Be strong, Bill.

Is the current strong?
Is the rock there firm?
Is either better
For me to be like?
What is my purpose?
Be strong, Bill.

Do all agree that strength is good?
Or that lack of strength is bad?
Cannot my weakness be a good?
Is there weakness in acceptance?
Is there peace in my acceptance?
Be strong, Bill.

So, what attitude to adopt?
Worry about how others judge?
For my relationship with cancer,
For my relationship with death?

And do I judge myself for it?
Be strong, Bill.

To understand this more deeply,
I need to fathom other words.
Like peace, purpose, and acceptance.
I need to choose my own purpose,
My solitary path to walk.
Be strong, Bill.

All these words to me seem hollow.
When first my eyes meet them,
They seem so good like a beacon,
They seem to resonate with light,
When truly they only lead to more words.
Be strong, Bill.

If peace can be strength for me,
Then I will accept strength only
Because my real beacon is peace,
Peace around me to allow me
To struggle just for understanding.
Be strong, Bill.

3. CHANGE
We resist it.
We deny it.
We guard ourselves
In fear of it.
Like it was the wolf and the terrorist.

And yet it is the only thing we can be sure of,

As sure as we are about the sun in the morning.
It is in our past and our present and the moment.
But the lack of variation in change also brings comfort,
As I learned to not rely on what I am used to.

I think back to other words, like to "Hope" and to "Strength."
Those eggshell foundation rocks that have falsely reassured us,
But not satisfied introspection, ye vile, vain words.
So we are left clinging to words that have no strength and
Fearing other words that in fact may bring inner peace.

Cancer changed me and others around on all sides.
Some get closer and others withdraw from my circle.
I deal with it every day, and, breath by breath, I learn it.
It teaches me patience and understanding and life,
While it saps my energy to fight, ending in peace.

So welcome change
And embrace it.
It will change me.
Enjoy the peace,
And understanding.

4. CURE

The Holy Grail,
The light at the end of the tunnel,
The daily dream,
The gift a person cannot earn.

Worth all the fighting,
Worth all the money,
Worth all the prayers,
Worth all the treatment.

The chemo,
The surgery,
The radiation.
The anything.

Illusive,
Misleading,
Deceiving,
False.

The label "cured" misleads.
It may come back,
Or another may come.
There are no promises.

There is no cure.
Five-year survival probabilities,
Remission, undetectable disease,
But not cure.

Scared

By Anonymous

I am not a writer nor do I have good grammar. But I would like to share something.

I am scared.

Not for myself, even knowing that I have MEN 2a, but I am scared for all of you.

I have never cried so hard as the day Rob passed away. He was just a man that took the time to meet my daughter at MDA and show her how concerned he was for her. I swear he left a hole in my soul the day he passed away. I'm scared to know that that will be my children's destiny (to die). I'm scared to read each and every one of your posts praying that you'll post a picture of your late night meals, and of your wife posting as Lori had to. You can edit the words in this and please don't share my name for both of my children are in this group and I, as their mother, have to be the strong one and not let them see the fear inside of me. I am just a simple lady with dreams of one day having answers to WHY ME????

A True Oxymoron That Comes With Cancer

By Elizabeth Carey

So what has cancer brought into my life? I've been pondering that question for a few months now, trying to find the right words to say, exploring those emotions I have so cleverly hidden. I've made countless attempts at writing things down on paper, only to re-read it and start all over again. I've tried to take myself back to the time when we first found out, examining those first emotions after hearing the words, "He has stage 4 cancer."

It's rather difficult for me. I've become so numb to all those feelings. In fact, some days I feel like I have no emotions left at all. But, first things first. I'm not a patient, and thus don't feel what it's like to have cancer in my body. I'm the spouse of a medullary thyroid cancer (MTC) patient, the "caregiver," so to speak, and thus I don't know what it's like to take a pill every day to replace a hormone my body needs. I have no clue as to the pain involved from surgeries to remove the bad stuff growing in my husband's body, or how the burn from radiation hurts so badly you can't sleep or eat for days. And last, but certainly not least, what it feels like knowing that it continues to grow and spread, and in the end there's little that can be done to stop it. I can only view it from the outside. I can only provide a different perspective and share what it's like to be the spouse whose husband has this incurable, awful disease.

I'm the caregiver. I'm the one who has to stand by watching someone I love as much as life itself battle this daily. I'm the one who gets to go to work, set it aside to stay sane, and keep the family going. I'm the one who gets to wonder why, wonder if a year from now—or two years, five years, ten—he'll still be with me. How long will I be able to say good night, I love you? How long will I see him when I come home at night and say good-bye in the morning as I head off to work? I get to see the ever-so-subtle winces of pain as I look into my husband's eyes, and although he really doesn't complain and he tries to hide it, I know he hurts somewhere inside because of the cancer. They say the eyes are the mirror of the soul, and as I look into his eyes I see how this disease has affected him, how it has affected us. For even though I'm not the patient and don't have the cancer growing inside me, I still get to live with this disease day in and day out. I get to see it take a toll on him, taking away little things here and there, stealing our future. It does something to you. It changes you, and causes you look at life so very differently. What is it? It's those lost dreams. It's the survival mode that you're forced into. It is cancer.

Being a caregiver is not something I ever aspired to be. It wasn't this world I'd chosen to join. It's a position that was thrust upon me, whether I was ready for it or not. When my husband was diagnosed three years ago I remember sitting in the hospital and listening to the surgeon telling us that he was going to die. There was no cure and no treatment for the kind of cancer he had, medullary thyroid cancer. I broke down in front of him then, the one and only time I did. I felt like my world was closing in around me as I watched those dreams we had for the future burst into flames. But when I looked at my husband all I could see was the sadness in his eyes. He looked so lost, so incredibly defeated. Like someone had just punched him in the gut and he was gasping for air. I had this overwhelming feeling of protection and love. I didn't want to hurt him. He was hurt already. He didn't need to worry about me. My job was to make sure he was okay and supported. A spouse, a caregiver.

So what is a caregiver, anyway? If you look up the definition online it will tell you it's a paid or unpaid position for a person who cares for someone with a medical or psychological disease or condition. But it's so much more than that. It becomes a way of life. When I go off to work in the morning, I go into the world of my profession. I focus on my teaching, working with my students and dealing with the world of higher education. When I come home I go into my caregiving role. Making sure my husband has eaten, seeing how he's feeling, asking what his day was like. I often feel torn between these two worlds. I have to try and maintain that balance on what I need to do at work, yet my husband and his needs are forever in the back of mind. It gets to be exhausting at times. I liken it to juggling balls in the air. I can't afford to drop one, or everything will come tumbling down.

Cancer has that way of taking things away from you, your stability, your sanity, your security. It takes away surprising things as well. With a diagnosis of cancer there are certain parts of your life you assume will be lost. I think everyone knows the toll it takes on the patient, the health issues it causes, and how most of the treatments can be worse than the cancer itself. But few people talk about the other things that cancer steals away from you. As the spouse of an MTC patient, I sometimes feel as though I no longer exist, that I have become invisible. I remember before cancer (or as I like to call it, B.C.), people would ask me how I was, how were the kids or the family? We were treated as a whole unit, all-important and part of the world. Now, they only ask about my husband, and that's where the conversation ends. It's almost like our children and I have ceased to exist. I certainly don't blame them for asking. Prior to this I would most likely have done the same, but cancer is an all-access disease. It not only affects the person with it, it also affects the entire family. People who don't live with it on a daily basis don't really think about it. They don't really understand. And while it's important to ask about the patient, it can be just as important to ask about the rest of the family. We are all still here and we're all dealing with the consequences of cancer, but cancer is not the only thing that defines us. Yes, I'm a caregiver to my spouse with cancer, but I'm also a wife and mother, a teacher and electrician by trade, a grandmother, a friend, a daughter, a sister, and now, apparently, a writer. I went from being a multi-dimensional individual to only having one significant characteristic. When my husband was diagnosed I lost all the various qualities of what made me the person I am, and now I'm merely an extension of my husband who has cancer. Our family unit has melted into the background. I think people tend to forget about the family and the impact it has on them. Not intentionally, it's just that their focus shifts. And the worst part about them asking about my husband is that nine times out of ten they don't really want to know. They are asking out of polite conversation and because that's what you're supposed to do. I think some of them want to know, but ultimately they're also afraid of the answer. I think in some respects it makes the mortality of the human condition too real. It makes them realize just how fragile life is and how quickly the tables can turn. However, as a person who is facing these circumstances on a daily basis, it's difficult for me to know what to answer. When I attempt giving them an honest answer, their eyes begin to glaze over and they get an almost panicked look in their eyes. The TMI look. If I lie and say everything is right with the world, they get this look of relief. Which one is the right way? I haven't a clue. The answer depends upon my mood, the day, and how my husband is feeling. Am I feeling nice and giving or am I feeling feisty and bitchy? This is definitely not something I would have thought about prior to the diagnosis.

Another loss along the same vein is that as a spouse and caregiver you also lose yourself in the sense that your days are no longer determined by how you feel. You become so entwined with your loved one. You begin to have your days determined by them. When my husband has a good day, I have a good day. When he has a bad day, so do I. It's not something you intentionally do, it's just what happens. When I think about our trips to the Mayo Clinic for his doctor visits every three months, it's no longer just he's going to the doctor, it has become we're going to the doctor. Once again, it's a subtle shift of the mind, but significant nonetheless. I don't know if it's the impact of losing myself from others' perceptions, or losing myself because of my own. Either way, it's not something I thought would happen, nor did I anticipate it when we first started this journey.

Then there's the loss of family and friends who start to disappear, especially after the initial diagnosis and treatment. Everyone gathers around when they first find out. People call all the time to check in and see how he's doing. Is there anything we need, etc.? Then slowly, one by one, they start to slip away. You hear from them less and less. I'm aware that life goes on, and as my husband continues to battle, the immediacy of the situation lessens. I also know, as time goes on, people have a more difficult time knowing what to say or do. But it's because time goes on that things become much harder. As the disease continues to spread, that's when you need the support of friends and family the most, and that's when it seems they disappear. I think the hardest part for me is my husband's family and their lack of support for him. We hear from them maybe every few months, and it's mostly the obligatory phone call. On my side of things, they've disappeared from my life almost completely. If I don't call them, I don't hear from them. They're oblivious to the reality of our existence. I try to understand their side of things. After all, they're losing a son, or sibling, and I know how it must be difficult. There's also that out of sight-out of mind that happens and a sense of denial that oftentimes will rear its ugly head. If you don't acknowledge it, it ceases to exist. But I see how much it hurts my husband when they don't call him or come by. I know they have lives, I know that their lives are not like ours, they don't face this every day where it's always in their faces, but I sometimes wish they had the ability to step into his shoes, into our shoes, and see how it feels. How there is an exclusionary part that comes with cancer. He isn't always up for long family gatherings, so yes, we sometimes decline. However, that doesn't mean we'll never say yes, and to stop even asking anymore definitely hurts. I honestly don't think it's done with a harmful intent. It's just another loss of cancer, a byproduct of the disease.

This leads me to the loneliness of cancer. There is the loneliness my husband feels at being the patient, and no one truly understanding his perspective. And there's the loneliness of being the spouse and no one understanding my perspective until they have actually been in my shoes. We've both been fortunate to have the meddie group to offset some of this. Reading about others' experiences and knowing that they, too, have felt these same things and know these same things, helps both of us a great deal.

But sometimes I need more. Cyber hugs can be great, but real ones are what you need at that moment. I've lost many friends through this journey. There are some who are still a part of my life but others have left. Our lives have veered off to different paths, and while they try and understand, they won't until, God forbid, they go through the same thing. The ones who are still around try and understand the best they can, but they have even told me that they don't know what to say, or what to do. I appreciate what they do try and do. I know they are attempting to support me in whatever way they can. But many try and "fix" the situation, when all I really need them to do is listen. I've been trying to not let cancer rule my life, and while there are days I can't help but think about it, I also try and live as normally as one can in a very abnormal situation. It still comes down to a lonely road to travel.

Lastly, for me there's a loss of emotion. At the beginning of our journey I was very emotional and would oftentimes go for a drive down to the river to cry alone. I felt an overwhelming fear of losing my husband then and couldn't even begin to look at the days or weeks ahead without sheer and utter panic. MTC was always present in my mind, and I'd wonder how many days we'd have left together. Part of this came from my husband's first surgeon, who informed us we needed to prepare ourselves for his death, and part of it was the cancer diagnosis itself, which seems to give a sense of urgency to living life quickly before it's taken away. I think I went through all the stages of grief back then, the sadness, the anger, the why did this happen to him, to us, why not me? And then the eventual acceptance of what is.

But as his cancer progressed, I discovered a whole new set of emotions that go along with a chronic illness. There's no way to prepare yourself for this, no manual to guide you. These emotions are different, not so immediate, much more subtle, and much easier to contain. Because my husband's cancer has continually progressed since his original diagnosis, there has never been that celebratory word called stable. He has never been stable. His tumors have never been stable. His numbers go up and down from various treatments, but the tumors continue to grow and spread. Eventually, my sadness—and for the most part, my anger—just went away. In fact, I pretty much became numb to it all. When you never get good news you learn to not anticipate it or feel disappointment. I think I closed away these emotions to protect myself and to help me stay strong. Unfortunately, in doing that I seem to no longer be able to get them back. I've become emotionally drained, and even when I should feel sad, or should cry, or should feel happy, I don't.

My father recently passed away. I was by his side as he died, holding his hand, and all my siblings were there, standing around. When he took his last breath, all my siblings began to cry and hug each other. I found I couldn't cry. I felt like I wanted to, tried to, but I couldn't. I know I should have. I should feel sadness and grief, but I literally felt nothing. I felt like I was dishonoring my father by my inability to do so, but I just couldn't. I don't know if it's because I've buried the emotions for so long in order to face each new challenge with my husband. Almost like a Pandora's Box, one that can't be opened, only it's my brain that holds the key. All I know is that I couldn't. I felt like I always did, numb. I loved my father very much. He was the one person who was there throughout this cancer journey for both my husband and me. My father died from complications of his cancer treatment and had taken care of my mother before she had died. He had that unique perspective of knowing both sides of the cancer equation, that of the spouse and caregiver, and that of the patient, but when I couldn't even cry at his deathbed I knew I lost something of true value.

This is perhaps the worst thing that cancer has taken away from me. I was even hoping that writing my story would help, but I cannot get there. The emotions are buried too deep. I've gotten so good at compartmentalizing my life and emotions in order to function on a day-to-day basis that I've lost a part of my humanity to this awful, crappy disease.

While I'd like to say that I've only *lost* things to cancer, I can't. I say this only because I hate the disease that much, and to give anything positive to it seems like a crime. But I honestly should say there have been some *positive* things that have come from this as well. I certainly wished it had not taken this for it to happen, but as with all things in life, both bad and good oftentimes comes from it. Cancer has given me a much truer sense of self. I've found that I'm much more focused in both what I want and also what I strive for. Prior to my husband's diagnosis I wasn't necessarily lackadaisical towards my future, but I wasn't necessarily laser focused on it, either. Prior to the diagnosis we'd made the decision that I'd focus on my career while he manned the home front. He had lost his hearing due to an unrelated condition, and along with the recession had lost his career. We made the decision at that time that I'd change my career and move into a less physically demanding job. I became the primary breadwinner of the family, and when we received his cancer diagnosis there was relief that we'd made the decision years before, because we were then not in a position of financial chaos.

With the cancer diagnosis, I've found a sense of urgency and a new focus on my career and what I want to attain. My husband has given me the strength, ambition, and support to continue to move up in my career and given me the ability to separate out parts of my life to maintain and achieve what I want. I've also gained confidence and strength from managing our lives with this disease. I suppose I always had those abilities, but the diagnosis and subsequent progression of his disease have given me that extra push I needed.

Another thing the cancer diagnosis has given me is my appreciation of life. There is truth in the statement to not sweat the small stuff, because in the end it really doesn't matter. Stupid little fights are too much work to have any value, and I don't have the energy or desire to really care about them. Those everyday things that I used to take for granted take on much more meaning. The feeling of his arms around me, the smile on his face, and saying I love you before going to bed. I've even learned to appreciate my husband's annoying habits. They used to bug the shit out of me, and while they still bug the shit out of me, I know there will come a time when I'll miss them terribly. When I began to face the fact that my soul mate would eventually be taken from me, I learned to appreciate everything about him and our day-to-day life. The changing of the seasons have new meaning to me because it's one more season to share, and I really don't know how many more I'm going to be given. I know that sometimes cancer will tear two people apart, but fortunately in our lives it has brought us closer together. I'm much more attuned to him now. We don't need so many words to say, but we can still talk for hours. I'm able to cherish these moments far more than I think I ever did. My husband tells me if it weren't for me he'd no longer be here. I am his rock and his reason for being. I don't think cancer necessarily gave us this, but we're now able to say the words and appreciate the moments more fully.

So in the end what has cancer brought into my life? Chaos, sadness, anger, love, gratitude, helplessness, and hope. It has altered my life in ways I never dreamed of. I often think about a quote from C.S. Lewis, "Experience: that most brutal of teachers. But you learn, my God do you learn." My experiences have shaped who I am, both good and bad, and I have continued to learn something from them. My part of the cancer journey with my husband has given me valuable experiences, with some sad losses along the way. In the end I'll try and remain grateful for each day I'm given with him, both the good and the bad.

Currently, my husband is facing the decision of whether or not to take the TKIs. I'll support him either way, but it also brings out my biggest fear of all. Losing him. It's my one deep dark secret: that I will not be strong enough to handle it in the end. That's the part that I'm scared of the most as his cancer continues to grow throughout his body. So, while I'll support his decision to not start the TKIs, I'll dread it as well, for without it he'll not survive.

In closing, I'll leave you, dear reader, with the following random thought: I'll continue to grieve as much as I will continue to hope. A true oxymoron that could only come with cancer.

I'm Still Here

By Michelle Wiley

Yes, I've been a bad blogger lately. I knew this day was coming and I've had to process all my feelings associated with it.

Before I can even begin to discuss this, I have to start with telling my story. This is the first time I've written it for the world to see. I still have the scar and will forever wear it proudly, I'm a survivor and here's my story.

In the summer of 2008, I had coworkers ask what was wrong with my eye. "Nothing", was my constant reply. It wasn't until then that I started actively paying attention to my eyes. Yep. The left one definitely was different from the right one. I mentioned this during an optometrist visit, and he promptly referred me to an ophthalmologist. After looking at numerous pictures and after two visits he decided my perceived eye problem was due to the way I was holding my head. Thankfully, he referred me to another ophthalmologist, who took one look and said it looked like I had Horner's Syndrome. Horner's occurs when there's damage to a sympathetic nerve. This can be attributed to a car wreck, open heart surgery, lung cancer, etc. I'd experienced none of these, so I had my first MRI. A couple of days later I got the call that there was an enlarged lymph node chain and a spot on my thyroid. I was told I might have lymphoma.

After frantic calls to my primary doctor and the ophthalmologist, I had an appointment with an oncologist, who ordered blood work, a

PET scan, and an MRI. I was relieved to hear I didn't have lymphoma. He referred me to a neurologist and an endocrinologist for the spot on my thyroid.

The neurologist ran several MRIs. There was still no reason for the Horner's. I was then referred to a neurological ophthalmologist. He advised it was a sporadic case of Horner's and was advised to keep an eye on it, and if it got worse and impeded my sight, I should come back in.

The endocrinologist advised me that most nodules were nothing. He left me with the decision to do nothing, have a biopsy, or have my thyroid removed. I decided to have the biopsy.

On January 9, 2009, I had the procedure, and it was awful. The procedure required taking three samples. I was warned that a preliminary reading would be taken to ensure they got enough samples. If not, I'd have to repeat the procedure. The shot to numb my throat didn't work. Not only did I feel the pressure of the ultrasound on my neck, I felt the needle go in, extract, and go out. Between each sample I laughed. It was easier for me to control my laughter than my tears. After the procedure I went back to work.

On January 11, 2009, Sam and I went to Vegas to celebrate my 30th birthday. We had a fabulous time, as always. In the back of my mind, I wondered about the results of my biopsy. I assumed no news was good news, so I didn't press it until I came back home.

Two weeks had passed since my biopsy without word about the results. I called the endocrinologist and was told to come in. If you know anything about hearing doctor's test results, most of the time they make you hear bad news in person. I rushed from work to the office. I couldn't find anyone to go with me. I went alone and heard the news that my biopsy was abnormal. In spite of hearing this, I tried to think rationally and logically. I looked to the endocrinologist for answers, but he was no help. I was told that basically I had to decide whether to have my thyroid removed or leave it.

I met with the otolaryngologist and scheduled my surgery on February 18, 2009, between semesters. I remember waiting and waiting to be prepped. Family was there keeping me company. The otolaryngologist told us he'd take out the enlarged lymph node chain and half of my thyroid. If it looked iffy, he'd take it all out. I requested that if he did, could someone please tell my family. He replied he would. In the middle of surgery a nurse talked to my mom and my brother, telling them they would take out all of my thyroid. When I was awakening from the anesthesia I had visits from the anesthesiologist and otolaryngologist. I thought I dreamt his telling me I had cancer.

On February 23, 2009, I was at home still awaiting the results. Mom had just gone to the grocery store to pick up some supplies. No doubt she was getting some of my favorite things. She always has spoiled me. I don't know what led me to call, but I did. I was told over the phone that I had Medullary Thyroid Cancer (MTC). An appointment was made to discuss everything and figure out our next steps.

I hung up the phone. Numb. Tears. No one to console me, since I was home alone. I called Sam, who at the time was coming back from Dallas. Kris answered the phone. I think I said, "Pull over. I have cancer." Sam talked to me for a bit. He assured me everything would be okay. He would come straight to my house. We would figure out a game plan, and he loved me.

The next call was to my brother, Russ. People who work retail often have crazy schedules. Thankfully, he picked up. I told him the news. After some comforting words he told me to be strong when I told Mom. It seemed like it took her forever to get home. She was happy when she came home. I hated to tell her. But I did and we both cried as we held on to each other. This whole day felt long and surreal. I did ordinary things, taking a shower, eating, having visitors. But everything was different.

On April 1, 2009, I had my second surgery to remove the rest of the lymph nodes in my neck and some in my upper chest. MTC spreads first to the lymph nodes and then to other parts of the body. It doesn't respond well to chemotherapy or radiation, so surgery is recommended. When talking about this with the surgeon, he advised that he'd use staples. I pleaded for him not to. He won. I remember looking at my neck for the first time. I cried. I looked like I belonged in a horror movie. I felt like I looked: awful. I was told that some other lymph nodes had enlarged since my first surgery, but like my first, they were benign.

There is so much after this part of the story. It involves me fighting with the insurance company to get my genetic testing. MTC can be sporadic or hereditary. Thankfully, my case was sporadic. Unfortunately, to this day I'm still fighting the insurance company regarding paying this claim. I don't want to bore you with this.

Thanks to God, I'm alive today. There are so many places in my story I could have dropped the issue with my eye or my thyroid. Most of the symptoms I had with MTC were attributed to other medical issues I have. Theoretically, I could still have it in me. Maybe I would have found out sooner, maybe later, when it metastasized into other areas, or never at all.

These thoughts and others I won't share often come to my mind. I don't think they'll ever leave. I struggle with being thankful. Sometimes I feel as though I am not thankful enough. With that being said . . .

Thank you. Chances are, if you're reading this, you've helped me. I remember the visits, the flowers, the cards, the talks, those who helped me shower, those who braided my hair, those who brought me comfort food, those who held me, those who let me cry. To this day I have a wonderful support system. Thank you. Thank you. Thank you. My battle has been won with your help. It's as much my victory as yours. I love you all.

May 1, 2015. It's been six years. Six. I'm truly one of the lucky ones. I was a Stage 1. When I go in for my yearly, I get a heaviness in my heart that remains until I get the results. I still struggle with being thankful. I still have dark thoughts too horrible to mention, and I still feel the love from friends and family. Throughout all this, I'm still here.

The Long And Winding Road

By Elizabeth Simons

My journey began in the summer of 2013. I went to see an allergist/immunologist for problems with my thyroid. His on-the-spot diagnosis of my Hashimoto's impressed me, and I thought he might be able to help me with my symptoms of sleeplessness and anxiety and a general feeling of jitteriness.

Dr. Pompous began with a round of tests. Then he ordered another round of tests. And then, guess what? Another round of tests. He never took action on any of the test results. He just kept testing, until I wondered if I'd have any blood left. He'd fold his hands prayerfully and recite one malady after another. It could be an adrenal tumor, or it could be a goiter, or it could be . . .

What? I asked. He'd shake his head and tell me we had to do more tests.

I finally got tired of his guessing game. He was looking for something rare and exciting, but I pointed out that maybe he should start wondering why I had a TSH of .008.

I went to an endocrinology clinic, where further testing revealed thyrotoxicosis, otherwise known as a thyroid storm. I was taken off my thyroid medications to allow my thyroid to heal.

I asked if I could have a couple of different dosages so I could adjust my medication in the future based on how I was feeling, especially as Hashimoto's has a way of going up and down. The department head was called in and scolded me severely for requesting such a thing. Dosages, she said, were strictly based on blood work.

Adios, I said.

I began to look elsewhere. I called three endocrinologists who served my area, but they were solidly booked. Finally, there was one left standing. I called his office and was able to get an appointment right away.

The decidedly dashing Dr. Smarty-Pants felt around my neck and ordered an ultrasound, which revealed a nodule on the right side. A fine needle biopsy showed I was positive for papillary thyroid cancer.

Cancer! I couldn't wrap my head around the word. I found out when Dr. Smarty-Pants' nurse called me. I thought she sounded a bit too chipper, given the nature of the news she was imparting. She said they'd made an appointment for me with a surgeon in their doctors' consortium. Hey, it was only papillary. What's the big deal?

Hey, it *was* a big deal! *She* wasn't the one with cancer.

And who was this surgeon, anyway? How many neck surgeries had he done? After talking it over with my husband, we decided we weren't going to have someone we didn't know cutting into my neck, given that there were things like major veins and arteries and nerves and vocal cords and stuff in there.

I called the cancer center at Barnes Jewish in St. Louis, and I had an appointment with an ENT surgeon/oncologist, Dr. Cut-Up, within a week. Things moved fast after that. I had my pre-op appointment, and was scheduled to have my thyroid removed a week later. Dr. Cut-Up had skills, and all went well.

Until the following week. At the post-op appointment Dr. Cut-Up informed me I didn't have papillary thyroid cancer after all. I had a very rare type of cancer known as medullary thyroid cancer, or MTC. I'd never heard the word, and really didn't hear what he was saying after that. I believe he told me I could go back home to have it treated, because it was just too far to drive.

Hey, wait. It wasn't too far to drive to St. Louis for surgery? Followed by, it's very rare but I'm supposed to find a local doctor with expertise in a rural area? He appeared perplexed and seemed very anxious for us to leave. So we left.

When I got home I had several messages from Dr. Smarty-Pants. Are you okay? How did things go? If I hadn't yet decided on a doctor for follow-up, could he be my doctor? How sweet, I thought.

He did some blood tests and a chest x-ray and a 24-hour urine collection. He looked at me with his carefully arranged look of concern and said, "You could have died during surgery, you know." Really? Good to know. I got the feeling he'd gone home and opened his diagnostic handbook and crammed his head full of facts about medullary thyroid cancer, triumphant in the secure knowledge that he was now an expert. And he was the only doctor in town with an MTC patient. Woo hoo!

Dr. Smarty-Pants then had his nurse make an appointment with the top-notch oncologist in their consortium. In fact, he was so top-notch that he was leaving in a month. "Excuse me, doctor," I said, "But what's the use in my having a work-up with someone who'll be gone soon, and then having to do it over again?"

I don't recall his answer.

Back home I turned on the computer and began searching. First, I found the ThyCa support group. Best thing I did. Then I looked for doctors and found one in St. Louis who was an MTC expert. Next best thing I did.

My initial thought was, what a shame I have to drive so far, followed by, "There's an expert in St. Louis and he's only three hours away? *Yes!*" I canceled the appointment with the local oncologist and made an appointment with Dr. Expert.

About this time I think I became more of a liability than an asset to Dr. Smarty-Pants. His bedside manner changed from conciliatory to exasperated. After all, I'd snubbed two of his colleagues. I was always asking questions, and I got the feeling there were things he just didn't know. Or he just didn't want to bother responding to. I'd send him articles, which he never acknowledged. I asked if the lab in his doctors' group followed the proper protocols for calcitonin testing, and he said, "I have no clue."

Really? Wouldn't the proper response be, "Let me look into this"?

The relationship was permanently severed when I asked him about a pain I was experiencing—because when you have cancer, you feel like everything's related to cancer—and his reply was a terse, "I can't be your PCP."

"Who said I was asking?" I replied.

I called another endocrinologist who had been highly recommended by a fellow meddie. At our local ThyCa meeting Dr. Splendid said I could contact her any time with my concerns, whether I was a patient or not. She treated the whole person, not just endocrine related symptoms. That clinched it. Dr. Smarty-Pants was history.

So now I have two good members on my team and feel very confident that I'm in good hands. I'm not so anxious. The MTC group encouraged me to always, always ask questions. Make sure my doctors are all on the same page. Keep records of everything.

Because in the end, I'm the one driving this bus.

My Thank You Note To Cancer

By Joyce Johnson

Not to give any of my power away, meaning I'm not lying down for this and certainly not giving up, but I'd like to thank cancer - more specifically, medullary thyroid cancer - for all that it has given and shown me.

Because of medullary thyroid cancer, or MTC, I now have a wonderful, beautiful extended MTC family. Never in a million years would I have been so fortunate to cross paths with so many amazing people. While every meddie has their own story to tell and their personal journey to travel, they all have one common denominator. They are all awesome! I guess that's one of the prerequisites. You must have a genetic mutation for awesomeness to get MTC. That's my story and I'm sticking to it.

Another thing that MTC has shown me is how giving and loving my husband and son are. Sadly, I've seen cancer divide and conquer in other families, but that's not the case for me. Not only have my wonderful husband and son stepped up for this challenge, so has my whole husband's family. In fact, I'll go on record saying I have the best mother-in-law *ever*. My nickname for her is FMIL, which stands for favorite mother-in-law. And trust me, those words are not hollow. I've had two previous mothers-in-law and she is hands down and leaps and bounds far superior. And I felt that way before I was diagnosed. So you can imagine how her loving and caring nature has elevated her in my eyes since my diagnosis. I can still see the tears well up in her eyes as we were sharing my news of cancer. But instead of turning into a shrinking violet, she instantly bounced back, encouraging me by saying, "If anyone can beat this, I know it's you."

Also, my husband has two brothers and one sister, who are all married with children, and I'm so blessed and happy to say each should be commended for their loving care and support. And I would be remiss if I failed to sing the praises of all my amazing friends. Every single friend has made themselves available to me and my husband, especially since cancer came into our lives.

I'd like to share a little story about how we came to adopt a bumper sticker as one of our life mantras. Shortly after I was diagnosed—as you might expect—we were a little down. Probably still in shock. As we were sitting in somber silence in traffic waiting for the light to turn green, I could feel Stanley's heart searching to find something to lift our spirits. And that's when he saw it: a bumper sticker. He gently coaxed me to look up and out the windshield to read what we now believe to be sage words. The bumper sticker stuck to the vehicle directly in front of us read as follows: *Cancer is my Bitch!* We could not believe it. Out of all the vehicles we could be sitting behind, it was that one with the perfect words we needed to see.

We give thanks to this day for that little miracle. It has kept a smile close to our lips and hearts and has certainly given us the gumption to carry on.

Respectfully, I say thank you to my cancer for showing me what an awesome life I have and what amazing family and friends I've been blessed with.

And don't forget, Cancer, you are my bitch.

One More Day With You

By Ashley Maderr

If a cancer patient falls
In love with you
Boy, let me tell you
Just how lucky you are.

Love from a girl who has seen death
While lying on the ultrasound bed,
Means the love that will withstand
All life's challenges, head-to-head.

Love from the patient in room 511
Who has undergone the surgery to save her life,
Is equivalent to the love of a newlywed bride
Who is still in awe of being your wife.

Love from someone who only survives
With the aid of treatment and pills,
Means love with all the strength
Her fragile little heart feels.

Because if a cancer patient
Falls in love with you
Man, you won't believe
Just what passion is yet to come.

Every ER trip will only break her heart
Because she knows you're trying to be brave,
Like how trips to the doctor are unspoken
In case one of you begins to cave.

Every minute alone with her will be rewarded
In sweet words with her affectionate smile,
As with your schedules and her worn out body,
These moments only come once in a while.

And every evening and every morning
You will see her eyes on you shining bright,
Praying and hoping for your well-being
So you can live longer and healthier than she might.

And now you know
When a cancer patient falls in love with you,
It means you are their chemo
And they will always fight their cancer.

For one more day with you.

All The Signs

By Anna Johnson

In 1993 my Dad died of thyroid cancer. Ten years earlier, when he was 54, a malignant supra clavicular node had been discovered and he had been diagnosed as having lung cancer and given four months to live. As far as I am aware he didn't even have a chest x-ray to confirm this erroneous diagnosis.

After about five years Dad developed a tumour on his spine and someone finally diagnosed thyroid cancer as the primary. There were no treatment options by then, so it was a case of a pretty awful downhill slide for the next five years, and then he was gone. There was no hint that there were different types of thyroid cancer, nor that there could be a familial element. I can only assume, as I was very much kept away from the detail, that no family history was ever asked for, as what I didn't know then, but do now, is that my paternal grandfather had also died of thyroid cancer at the age of 52.

Fast forward to 2008. One morning as I smoothed moisturizer into my neck I thought I could feel a lump in the right side of my throat, so off I went to my trusty GP. I told her that my Dad had died of thyroid cancer, and that my granddad had also died of some kind of cancer in his throat - both of them at an early age. I was 46 years old at the time. The GP examined my throat, smiled indulgently, and informed me that what I could feel was (and for some reason I remember this as if it were yesterday), "a perfectly natural asymmetry of the voice box". I left, relieved.

Nine months later I was back again, asymmetry of the voice box still there, but this time a bit painful, which had renewed my concerns. Another examination. "Nothing there, but your throat's a bit red. It's just a minor infection. If the pain is no better in a couple of weeks come back." The pain went - that bit obviously was an infection. I didn't go back. I learned to live with an asymmetrical larynx!

In 2013 I had some unpleasant abdominal symptoms, which I put down to the approaching menopause. I went to (a different) GP. For some reason, and thank goodness for this, she decided to do a CEA test, which can show as a marker for bowel cancer. She phoned me 2 days later to tell me it was "a little elevated" (56!), and could I come back so she could talk to me about a colonoscopy. I couldn't believe I could have bowel cancer - I just didn't think I had the right symptoms - so I started looking up information about CEA. I found it was also a marker for a form of thyroid cancer that could be passed down genetically. I felt cold and shaky. I felt my "asymmetrical larynx". I looked at my father's and grandfather's death certificates. I told my GP I didn't need a colonoscopy, because I was pretty certain I had Medullary Thyroid Cancer.

Two days later, on 13 September 2013, an ultrasound confirmed that I had a lump in my thyroid. So, father and grandfather dead from thyroid cancer, CEA of 56, lump in the thyroid. (No, the larynx was fine, since you ask - no one even commented on its strange shape). Now, I'm just an accountant, but I'd managed to work out that the chances of me having MTC were around 99.99%. Nevertheless, there seemed to be a whole battery of tests I needed to go through to confirm this. I do understand that the histology stuff is necessary, that you need a baseline calcitonin reading, and that you need a pre-surgical catecholamines and metanephrines test. What I don't understand was why you have to wait 3 weeks for the results of each of these tests, and you can't seem to have them in parallel, but have to wait for one set of results before the next test can be undertaken. So, I didn't get my surgery until 18 November, by which time my blood must have been almost pure Valium and red wine!

I was lucky that the first consultant I saw recognized that I needed to be referred to a specialist centre. It's just a shame he wasn't the specialist, as he remains the only medical professional throughout my MTC experience who has treated me as an individual, one who has a brain, but is also, justifiably I feel, shitting herself.

I was referred to one of the flagship British cancer hospitals, the "Royal Marsden". There, I have generally been treated as one of the following:

- a know it all
- a pathetic little child
- a worry guts
- a person with far too many questions
- a fucking nuisance.

I had a TT and selective right neck dissection. 38 lymph nodes were removed, and all were negative for malignancy. My calcitonin one month after surgery was undetectable. I drank champagne and bought a very expensive coat, and tried to be optimistic. All the news I was getting was as good as it could possibly be under the circumstances. I was T2 N0 M0. Stage 2. Totally curable apparently.

At this stage I believed I had had an excellent surgeon. All the "reports" suggested this to be the case. He seemed to be revered. I was amazed to find that my surgery took just two and a half hours. Other people seemed to be suffering much longer surgeries. I had been lucky here, hadn't I?

And yet... I couldn't stop the nagging voice that said there must be rogue cells circulating, waiting for a later chance at killing me. After all, I had suffered a five-year delay in diagnosis. This surely was not good news. Also, the pathology report seemed to my amateur eyes to suggest that my tumour was perilously close to the edge of my thyroid, and this frightened me. According to my specialist surgeon and my specialist oncologist, though, these issues posed *no* problem. All that mattered was that there was no spread beyond the thyroid, undetectable calcitonin, blah, blah, blah. I wanted to know why there appeared to be a difference in the ten-year survival statistics between stage 1 (100%) and stage 2 (93%) - surely I might have been a stage 1 five years earlier and therefore have had a better chance of survival? My questions have always been dismissed - never answered. Perhaps they don't have answers, but I wish someone would admit that, rather than treat me so patronisingly. All they would say to me, over and again, was that the chance of my cancer coming back after it had been caught at such an early(?) stage was VERY small, and I should stop worrying about it.

A year after my surgery I noticed a small lump on the right side of my neck. I mentioned it at my check-up. They said it was just a normal lymph node, but that they would do an ultrasound to put my mind at rest. I asked why it had suddenly made an appearance. There didn't seem to be an answer to that one either. Anyway, it was too small on the ultrasound to see all the features clearly, so they did another one six weeks later, and said it looked fine. Calcitonin still undetectable, but anxiety on the rise!

In February 2015 my husband and I went to India for 8 weeks. We spent the first two weeks touring Rajasthan and the next six weeks in Kerala, a favourite place for us. We have friends there now and it feels like a second home. This year my lovely American friend, who lives in Kerala, introduced me to his yoga teacher, and we had great fun doing yoga together on my friend's roof terrace. This teacher was amazing. I made so much progress with him, especially after having felt heavy and lethargic for so long. He was also a superb masseur. By the time the holiday ended I had loads more energy, my body shape had improved, I felt stronger and happier, my lower back pain had gone, and....my cellulite had all but disappeared! This man was serene and calm and made me feel safe, confident and happy. As far as I was concerned he had almost magical powers, and I felt as though nothing bad could happen to me all the time I was there. I wanted to stay forever. Oh, did I mention that he is young and heart-stoppingly beautiful? Actually, I felt young and beautiful too. And I noticed that my first thoughts in the morning and my last thoughts at night were not about MTC, but about all the things I wanted to do, and how happy I felt. In the last year and a bit I had forgotten about happiness and enthusiasm, and plans.

When I got home I was determined to continue with my yoga progress, and I wanted to work on looking and feeling better generally. I had got a taste for it. I felt as though I had a future where unexpected and exciting things, and achievements, were possible again.

One week after my return I went for my blood tests. For the first time since the nightmare began I didn't cry when they took my blood. Two weeks later I went for my check-up. My neck was examined and declared to be fine. My CEA was undetectable. The calcitonin results were still awaited. (Why they take three weeks to come through is beyond me - it's excruciating).

One week later I phoned for the calcitonin results. No longer undetectable. Low (2.2), but no longer undetectable. It felt like some kind of awful film. It was all going so well, and then.

So, it appears I am not "cured". I doubt I will live a normal lifespan. Maybe I won't even get ten decent years. At diagnosis I was distraught and I knew that I would spend the rest of my life looking over my shoulder, but I did have hope of a cure. All the "experts" told me that was highly likely. Now I am struggling a bit with the hope thing. I feel desperately cheated and let down. Perhaps my operation was so much quicker than everyone else's because it wasn't thorough enough. Perhaps my "experts" aren't expert enough. Perhaps I'm an experiment.

I now know that MTC spreads early and microscopically. I don't know that because a doctor told me. I know it because I read it on the internet. So, no problem with the five-year delay in diagnosis then! I know from the internet that if calcitonin has been undetectable, and then increases, that this is "highly suggestive" of a recurrence. Is it a good thing or a bad thing that we can track this horrible disease so accurately, and yet do nothing, in the long run, to cure it?

Perhaps there just aren't enough of us to make a cure profitable.

So now I have to go for another ultrasound, and a repeat calcitonin test. And then what?

I know I need to let go of my anxiety and my anger, but I am struggling with how to do this.

So, I am reading inspirational stories of others determined to make the best of life and do all the things they want to while they can. And, of course, "while they can" may be a long time with MTC. So it's just silly to waste that time being cross and worried. I am still alive and, as my fabulous husband will confirm, kicking.

We're going back to Kerala in the New Year. Somehow it makes me feel more spiritual, even though I have no religious belief whatsoever. I think spirituality aids acceptance. And I will be doing yoga with my lovely friend. And did I mention that the yoga teacher is heart-stoppingly beautiful?

Medullary Thyroid Cancer Is Not A Blessing

By Dara Michelle Hoffman

I'm not sure where or how the rumor started that cancer was a gift.

But if you ask me, it's a gift from hell and a gift that keeps on taking. Taking people I love away and slowly taking bits and pieces of me.

The darkness is at times more than I can bear. I sometimes think the loneliness and grief will swallow me whole. But I'm here, and I persist. Some days a dark cloud of fatigue follows me, with accompanying aches and pains, lumps and bumps, as I cling desperately to "normal." The challenge is that I *look* normal. In fact, I look better than normal, and I do an Academy-Award winning job of acting normal. But inside I'm sad and scared, and asking: Why Me? Why did I get cancer? Was it environmental exposure? Was it my years of an unhappy marriage? How did this happen to me? Why did this happen to me? I shouldn't ask, I shouldn't wonder.

But I do.

I don't just wonder about me. I wonder about how this happens to so many people I love, and sometimes I wonder how or why I outlive them. Is it faith? Is it confidence? My belief in miracles? The herbs I take? I know it's probably just dumb luck that I get to live another day. Don't get me wrong. I'd try anything to get this shit out of my body. I've tried: turmeric, asparagus, gallons of alkaline green juice,

Chinese herbs, Reiki, lymphatic trampoline, infrared sauna, a vegan diet, a vegan raw food diet, a low carbohydrate diet, mindfulness. And yes, enemas. Coffee enemas, to be exact. I have an arsenal of herbs and off-the-market prescriptions, including Naltrexone and dichloracetate (DCA).

I want to live, and ironically, I'm a mental health therapist who works with clients who want to die. Oh, the *irony*! The irony that I, a *certified health nut*, have *cancer*.

The one thing I ask of you is please *don't* blame me. I beat myself up enough, and think of how much I have lost: loss of energy, loss of motivation and the depression that is always lurking. Since diagnosed with cancer, the world looks so different. I try to not sweat the small stuff. Life has to be more than just paying bills.

I cherish the moments with my children, and when I watch my daughter dance, my heart soars.

I also had to face the nagging truth that I was in an unfixable marriage, and if cancer didn't get me then I was certain my unhappy marriage would suck me up and spit me out. I also was spreading myself too thin trying to balance my career and motherhood. I've had to make major life changes in my job and personal life. No time to waste. And so cancer has given me overwhelming fear and unrelenting courage at the same time.

What do I have to lose by speaking and living my truth?

The gifts of cancer are gratitude and humility. I have gained a sensitivity and kindness I did not know before. I am more non-judgmental and my empathy breaks my heart wide open. I don't have time to waste on fighting (not that I'm perfect). I only have time for living and loving. I want to watch my daughter dance and my son dazzle me with his quick wit. I want to sweat, savor each bite, taste the bitterness of emotional pain, and the sweetness of romantic connection. Because living like this is far better than the alternative. I'm humbled and grateful for each sleepless night. I now see the love around me was always there because I'm now less busy with unimportant activities.

I only have today, and some days I have no energy and I want to give up and give in. But the sun always *does* come up tomorrow, even in Oregon. And whenever I can't make sense of how or why this happened I look at my dog and her unconditional love. She doesn't see cancer. She sees me, and she loves me for just who I am. When I'm sad she draws near. When I'm tired she gives me space, and she encourages me to get up and off my butt and go for a walk outside. She makes me realize I am not defined by cancer. It's just one aspect of my complicated and beautiful life.

I have formed the most compassionate friendships with my fellow cancer sisters and brothers. I have witnessed empathy from unexpected colleagues. I have seen a love from my family I would not have known existed. And I have learned to accept help when I lie flat on my face, nose on the ground. I now know when I sink down that dark hole if I can't get out, someone will help me out, and if not, my dog will hang out as we wait out the storm.

So please, if you understand one thing, cancer is not a gift. It is not something I drew to myself for a higher spiritual process. I'm not stronger then you. I'm not a warrior in the battle for my life. It's just a screwed-up cellular breakdown whose mystery I wish I could unravel. And if I did know the reason why—not enough green juice? Too much past and present life trauma? Or the dumb luck of growing up near a nuclear power plant that unleashed chemical toxins on innocent people—does it really matter?

This disease is a part of me. I accept it and I want you to, as well. All I want is what you want, a life full of love, friendship, family and peace. Instead of fighting for it, I surrender.

So please know that even on my darkest days, I love you and I thank you for just being *you*.

How Cancer Upended My Life—And Gave Rise To A New One

By David Kalish
Author of *The Opposite of Everything*

Three weeks before my wife and I were to move to Mexico City, where a coveted job promotion awaited me, my doctor phoned me with results from my latest CT scans. My cancer had spread to my lungs. He suggested I see an oncologist right away. He suggested one on Long Island.

I let the phone go silent. It was May 2000, and my excitement over the new job, Latin American correspondent for The Associated Press, had been building for months. I'd taken months of intensive Spanish. My wife Ingrid and I had sublet our apartment in Brooklyn, changed our AP health insurance from domestic to international, sold our car, and put a deposit on one in Mexico. We'd gotten married just weeks earlier so Ingrid, a Colombian doctor on a student visa, could travel freely across borders with me. I didn't want to be without her.

Now everything felt shaky. Sucker-punched by the news of spots in my lungs, I placed the phone in its cradle and fell back into the couch. *Why now?* Now was the time for me to pack my clothes, not visit a new doctor. I badly wanted to move past my diagnosis of Medullary Thyroid Cancer six years earlier and my three neck operations, which left me with a permanently hoarse voice. Despite everything, my cancer had seemingly stayed confined to my neck. I wanted nothing more than to plunge into normality and stretch into new areas that challenged me, helped me grow.

Instead I felt like the butt of some cosmic joke. When I told Ingrid about the multitude of spots in my lungs, each smaller than one centimeter, she was unequivocal. "You need to see the oncologist as soon as possible," she said, flipping through Yellow Pages. But I responded with defiance.

"How am I going to squeeze in another doctor's appointment?" I protested, thinking I could just get treated in Mexico. "We're moving 3,000 miles in two weeks!"

Let me tell you something about Ingrid. My second wife, she's a self-directed, headstrong woman. As a native of war-torn Colombia, she'd watched her father die in a hospital, the victim of a carjacking, and fled the violence of her home country to make it as a doctor in America, barely knowing English initially. In contrast to my first wife, who had a tough time coping with my diagnosis, Ingrid married me knowing full well I had cancer.

"Well you have fun in Mexico," she said. "I wish you the best."

"You mean *we'll* have fun."

"You either take care of yourself, or be alone," she said firmly, fingers stopping on the phone number of the oncologist on Long Island.

Her thin smile told me she wasn't kidding. Seeing I had little choice, two days later we drove from Brooklyn to the doctor's clinic in Great Neck. His office was lined with floor-to-ceiling walls of diplomas and certificates and honors. He immediately made me feel tense, presumptively encouraging me to "think of me as your quarterback." After listening to my lungs, he let his stethoscope go slack and had my wife and me sit across his big desk.

He said my breathing sounded clear - for now - and suggested I start a regime of chemotherapy in three months.

"Chemo as in where?" I said, not caring how stupid the question sounded.

"Why here in my clinic, of course," he said. "Where we can keep a close eye on you and monitor side effects and mix up the recipe, if needed."

"Why don't you just give me the recipe? I'll just find a doctor in Mexico City, see what he thinks, and get treated there."

Ingrid kicked me under the chair, whispering: "David, you're not cooking tamales here!"

The doctor cleared his throat. "I wouldn't recommend moving to a developing country at a time like this. You should focus on getting well. Your lungs sound clear but one day you could be battling for breath. My goal is to delay that day as long as possible - but I can't do it without you here."

Ingrid and I argued about it when we returned to our car. Instead of turning the key in the ignition, I spoke my mind. "Don't you understand? This is my dream! Just like when you came up to the United States to study medicine. You came here to succeed, and I'm going to Mexico City to succeed as a foreign correspondent. Following my dream is probably the best thing I can do for my health."

"I didn't risk my life trying to succeed. I didn't have pulmonary metastases and move to the air pollution capital of Latin America."

Not just lung spots, but pulmonary metastases. That's what she called them. The medical phrase weighed on my nerves, underscoring the seriousness of my condition. We argued about it some more when we got home but I knew it was hopeless. Much as I didn't want to admit it, Ingrid - not just my wife, but also a doctor - made sense. I needed to focus on getting better, instead of learning a whole new language and job in a strange country, because nothing else mattered if I didn't.

The next few weeks blurred past in a daze. I felt like a marionette jerked around by a puppeteer, with no control over his destiny. I informed the subletters they couldn't, after all, have my apartment, bribing them with $2,000 so they wouldn't sue me for breach of contract. I switched back our health insurance from international to domestic. I canceled the movers. I forfeited my $350 deposit on a car in Mexico and scanned the classifieds for a used one in Brooklyn to replace the one I'd sold. I settled back into my position on AP's international desk, editing overseas stories by reporters stationed in exotic places that reminded me, painfully, of the one I'd given up.

My career setback was just one of many tests thrown at me by my cancer's spread to my lungs. An equally daunting challenge came a week later when we met with the oncologist to set up my treatment schedule, which started in three months.

"Before we start," he told Ingrid and me, "you should know that chemo can damage the sex cells. I suggest you visit a sperm bank. Or try to make a baby the natural way."

I nearly burst out laughing. "Oh, a fantastic idea. Let's make a baby!" I pictured myself running around, bald and nauseous and career-emasculated, chasing after a kid with a leaky diaper. It would be my ultimate humiliation.

But no one else laughed. "It's settled," Ingrid said brightly

"Just do it," the doctor said, quoting the Nike slogan, nodding in agreement.

"This is happening way too fast!" But my protests rang hollow to a woman who once regularly delivered babies in a Bogotá hospital. Newborns practically leapt with gratitude into her waiting hands, she once said. Ingrid argued it could be our last chance to bring our progeny into the world. Consider the children who might never eat guanavanas, watch the sea lions in Prospect Park, or eat dim sum in Chinatown. Consider children who might never be born let alone have children of their own. "Now do you see, David?"

I foresaw my own defeat and resigned myself to yet another sacrifice on my road back to health. Maybe I'd get lucky: it took the average couple far longer than just a few months of trying to get pregnant, so perhaps we'd fail to conceive prior to the start of my chemo. I could only hope.

But wouldn't you know it? Ingrid and I were successful right away. And not just that. Roughly three months after conception - the day after my first treatment - my symptoms crashed head-on with my wife's morning sickness, compounding my misery.

I woke up that morning, listening to the awful whir of my portable fanny pack pumping chemo through a tube into my chest. My stomach churned, threatening to work its way up, and I turned to ask my Ingrid to hand me my anti-nausea pills from the night table. But she wasn't around. Too desperate to wonder why, I staggered to the bathroom and made a beeline for the toilet. I hurled. Just then Ingrid teetered in, looking as sick as I felt. As if to demonstrate the correct method, she vomited too, but neatly and quietly, like the Queen of England might pour tea. She wiped her lips with a tissue, and dabbed Crest on her toothbrush.

"Do me a favor and vomit more softly," she said, after gargling. "I don't want to hear your inner pig. You don't know how sick I feel."

"But I think I do," I said weakly, in no mood to sympathize.

As if on cue, my gut spasmed again, at the same time a loud bark escaped me, like a seal during feeding time at the zoo.

Ingrid shook her head in disappointment and left the bathroom. I flushed the toilet, unsure where this nightmare was leading. The last thing I frankly needed in my delicate state was retching lessons from a pregnant woman.

As the weeks progressed, our symptoms further converged, and I grew afraid the stress of coping with my cancer would come between us - much as it had dragged down my first marriage. A few days later, I spied a clump of hair in the shower drain. Examining it closely, I determined it was mine. As I dried myself with a towel, feeling emasculated and shaky, Ingrid strode up. Rolling up the bottom of her shirt, she revealed seven wiry black hairs sprouting under her naval. She showed me her upper neck, where fresh fuzz clung to the underside, and told me she sadly felt like an old lady now.

"Whoop-di-doo," I said, showing her the hairball. "Thanks to chemo, I've got a clump."

She stared at me as if discovering gold. "First we share stomach problems. Then you lost hair; I gained hair in new places. Don't you see? We're becoming opposites, but in a similar way!"

She smiled in a way that creeped me out and touched my patchy scalp as if to share her new sense of solidarity with me, but I nudged her away. I wanted to cling onto what I still had of my hair - and my dignity. I was in no mood to celebrate.

"Please don't touch," I said. "It's very delicate."

"If your hair bothers you so much, let me shave you. Lots of sexy men are bald. Bruce Willis. Agassi. There's no need to look like a bad lawn."

"Sure, go ahead," I snapped, thinking of a barbershop from *Village of the Damned*. "But first let me shave your peach fuzz."

She glared at me. "So it will grow back as stubble? Like a man with - how do you say? - five o'clock shadow? It's enough I feel like an old lady with fuzz. You're certainly not helping!"

She left the bathroom upset, leaving me to think things over. I felt like a bad man with bad hair. Not to mention a bad stomach. It wasn't so much I didn't sympathize with her. It's just that my own suffering left me less tolerance to cope with hers.

We went several days without talking much. I thought back to how cancer had spread like a virus through my first marriage. Little conflicts with my wife grew into big ones. I worried the same thing could happen again. I imagined Ingrid's pregnancy hormones swimming inside her blood in tempo with the chemicals eroding my insides. I researched her condition over the Internet. "Human chorionic gonadotropin," I learned, helped nourish the fetus by diverting nutrients from the mother's bloodstream, provoking nausea. My finding reminded me that Ingrid recently had cut down on eating. A typical meal for her was a couple of sweet rolls, maybe coffee. *Shouldn't pregnant people eat twice as much, instead of half?* I pictured our bony nascent child locked in a moist pinkish room, jittery as a puppy lapping espresso.

Paternal protectiveness flickered on and off inside me, and stayed on for a while. I began to worry more about the growth inside of her than the one in me. One evening from the hallway I spied her lying on the bed, where she'd taken to spending hours each day, Spanish soap opera on the TV. She was tear-streaked, hands resting on her bare swollen stomach. "*Mi bebe,*" she said softly. "*Mio.*" My baby. Mine. I heard nurturing and loneliness in her voice, as if only she cared for this unborn child. I felt an urge to give her a hand. I read up in a book about natural remedies for morning sickness. One day I carried a tray of cubed tofu and a glass of vinegar into the bedroom.

"Are you feeding me *dice*?" she said, face tensing over the small white cubes.

"Would you prefer a sip of warm vinegar?"

She fiddled with the tofu knife, prompting me to back up a few inches. "Let me help you," I insisted. "Our child needs to eat and you, my dear, are the only restaurant in town."

"Maybe feed her something Colombian instead," she said. "Now you know how I feel when I wanted to shave you. It is my body. I cannot tell my body to want something it doesn't - the same way you stopped me from helping yours."

That night, I had a nightmare about lump reversal - Ingrid birthing a tumor, and a fetus surgically removed from my throat. I jerked awake, famished and nauseous, squinting into the low morning sun through the window. I left Ingrid sleeping in bed, her back to me like an icy fortress, put on a baseball cap over my patchy scalp and went outside to forage for food that wouldn't make me gag.

My first stop was at a café on Park Slope's Seventh Avenue, where I ordered a cappuccino, but after one sip I spilled it down a sewer grate. When I gazed up, I saw I stood in front of a bodega, overripe platanos displayed in bins. An idea came to me. I went inside and bought a loaf of Bimbo, a crunchy bread Ingrid once told me she liked. Returning to the apartment, I showed her it and uttered the only four-syllable Spanish word I knew: "*Mantequilla?*" Butter?

She seemed too stunned to answer; I brought a stick of butter from the kitchen and spread some across a slice for her. Shutting her eyes, she crunched down.

She blinked as if waking from a dream. "Wait till I tell my mother you're feeding our child Colombian food!" She crunched some more. "I remember toast for breakfast every Sunday in my home. And the fruits! In Colombia, the papayas and guanabanas so ripe and sweet and large." A tear slipped down her cheek as she ate a second slice, rambling on with nostalgia.

"You are eating," I whispered, happily. Struck with empathy, I handed her a razor. Her face lit up. She pulled me to the bathroom, ran the water warm, splashed it across my scalp, and sprayed foam from her leg-shaving kit into her hands. For the next twenty minutes, as she hummed a Colombian melody, she spread foam and stroked the razor across my patchy skull, tracking its bumps and lumps gentle as a mother bird preening its fledgling.

"*Gracias,*" she said, when she was done, admiring her handiwork. "I felt I was living with a sick person. Now you're almost sexy."

Taking a deep breath, I gazed at my reflection and touched my smooth glistening skull as if it were someone else's - someone cool with the situation, not angry and bitter over it. I realized something about Ingrid. *She needs to nurture her sick husband, because if she can, her helpless unborn child should be a cinch.*

The unspeakable tension in me lifted a bit. I imagined my lump having a one-on-one conversation with hers, breaking the communications barrier. A tête-à-tête, perhaps. "Maybe," I joked, "we can get a group rate on lumpectomies."

She kissed my scalp. "Please don't refer to our future child as a lump."

I wasn't done paying my dues, staying bald and nauseous for the duration of her pregnancy. It turned out, after all that, the chemo didn't do much except make me feel sick. The spots in my lungs kept growing. But five months later I got my money's worth. Ingrid gave birth to a healthy eight-pound girl named Sophie, and I felt, in a sense, that I'd given birth too.

At night in our Brooklyn apartment, Sophie would curl up in Ingrid's arms, and I'd gaze at the two of them sleeping like peas in a pod. If it ended with this tiny kid asleep, face scrunched against my wife's milk-swollen bosom, I was cool with that. Because she wouldn't have been born if my wife and I had gone on to Mexico. Sure, we might have had children, but they wouldn't be Sophie, who would grow into a gifted artist, pianist, and a kind friend, and become my constant reminder, day in day out, of why I needed to carry on to the best of my ability, no matter what life throws my way.

And I did. After giving up chemo, I entered a clinical trial for a novel cancer drug, Caprelsa, with fewer side effects, that today holds my Medullary Thyroid Cancer at bay. Sophie had her Bat Mitzvah last year, and we live in a spacious house in upstate New York instead of the cramped fourth-floor walk-up in Brooklyn where we used to live. Summers, we sow seeds in a little garden plot, weed tomato plants, and set down aluminum pie plates filled with Budweiser to drown the slugs. My novel, a fictional account of my cancer journey that ends with Sophie's mikvah, was published last year after gestating for thirteen years in the womb of my mind.

In retrospect, cancer tore up my life - and gave rise to a new one. Maybe the puppeteer pulling my marionette strings didn't do such a bad job, after all.

Running Rampant

By Joyce Johnson

The day I was diagnosed with MTC started out like any other day. The only difference was I had a doctor's appointment at 8:00am for an annual physical. I thought by having an early morning appointment I would miss less work that day.

Boy was I wrong.

As my doctor was just about to finish with my physical exam, he stepped behind me to replace the otoscope back into the wall charger. According to him my ears looked fine. While he was still behind me, he reached around and touched my neck. I came up off that exam table like he had stabbed me in the neck. Seriously, the pain was so severe it brought tears to my eyes. I asked him why he thought it necessary to knife me. All big eyed, he said, "I promise I didn't knife you." Long story short, he sent me for an ultrasound of my neck. So, instead of heading to work, my husband and I went to the closest radiological center for me to get the ultrasound done.

About mid-day we arrived at work and didn't think much more about what had happened that morning. Then a couple of hours later I received a call from my doctor's office asking me to come back to the office to have more blood drawn. They were very insistent saying just, "Be here before 4:30pm today, because we have a courier waiting to take your blood to a special lab". I said, "Ok", and hung up the phone. Then I called my husband, asking him if he could get away from work and come pick me up to return to my doctor's office. Without hesitation he said, "Of course".

It felt strange returning to my doctor's office. I could feel every eye trained on us as we were escorted back to an exam room. This was the first time we had ever been "fast-tracked" to be seen by my doctor. I remember thinking, this is what a real life Monopoly game must feel like. We passed go and paid a lot more than $200.00 in the end. Anyway, my husband and I had a sinking feeling that something very serious was going on. Within a couple of minutes my doctor walked in and honestly, I felt sorry for him. The paper in his hand was rattling from his hand shaking uncontrollably. It was a steady tremble. So, even before he gave us the news, we knew. Although, I tried to fill the room with idle chatter, thinking if I could keep my doctor from talking I would have one more second, one more minute of being cancer free. But, my doctor cut me off, saying, "I have some test results here".

I cut him off by saying, "I've told you all along that thyroid issues run rampant in my family."

He trumped me by saying, "this is way worse than running rampant".

It was then that he explained that he wanted to re-run the calcitonin test to confirm there was no lab error. We had no idea what a "calcitonin" was. He went on to say that he had already made some phone calls and made an appointment for me to see an endocrinologist. He said normally there is a six month waiting list to see this endo, but due to my circumstances he was able to get me in first thing Monday morning. Just when I thought our world couldn't sink any lower, hearing the urgency in his voice took away any hope that there could be a mistake. Anyway, Monday came and we stopped by to pick up the packet of new test results from my primary doctor and we made our way to see this highly recommended endocrinologist.

Registering was a blur. It was only when I was lying supine on his exam table that I really came to realize that fine needle aspirations hurt. He did no fewer than eight and no more than twelve sticks. All that I clearly remember were the forty eight slides he made from the fluid he sucked out of my neck. He was meticulous about making sure the stains on the slides were perfect before he asked an assistant to box them up and send them off to the lab.

My husband and I are known for being big talkers, which is why we asked a million and one questions. Unfortunately, we never felt sated with any of the answers. Secretly, I think there was a part of us that thought maybe if we don't research on the internet then maybe it won't be as bad. But, on the other hand, we felt maybe we could be empowered by gathering as much information as humanly possible from these doctors. Needless to say, we were in a constant struggle of what was the best way to proceed. Early on, the most frustrating thing was not being able to truly connect with my highly recommended endocrinologist. It was only after I pressed him to provide answers that we found out he really had no more experience with MTC than the next guy. At that point in time we didn't know he had none. It turns out my primary doctor had the most firsthand experience and knowledge from his residency and internship done twenty years prior at M. D. Anderson.

My primary doctor and my endocrinologist put their heads together and made the executive decision on which surgeon I should see. We spent the days leading up to my big cancer surgery running to and from a whole host of other medical tests. As it turns out, my body was presenting with other questions that the experts felt needed answering in a timely manner, as well. Maybe that's why we let some of the "research" fall by the way side. Or maybe I'm making excuses for letting unanswered questions go. But I'm here to say the stereotactic breast biopsy rivaled the pain of the fine needle aspirations I'd had done only days before. It's true we had a lot going on but looking back I'm inclined to think we should have educated ourselves more. The only reason I'm giving us a pass on this is because I've found nothing good comes from second guessing oneself or having regrets.

Finally, the day arrived and I was heading into my cancer surgery. It had been explained that I would be having a combination of surgical procedures. It was a mouthful to say the least. I had a total thyroidectomy, a modified radical right neck dissection followed by a central compartment chest dissection. All total the surgery was just shy of nine hours and when I came out, I looked as if I was on the losing end of a fifteen round fight with none other than Muhammad Ali back in his prime. Originally, I was scheduled to be in the hospital for no more than a day, two days tops. However, six days later I was finally released. To this day, I still have after effects resulting from the surgery, but knowing what I know now, I'm not complaining. I believe the surgeon did the best he could with what he had to work with.

I found out after it was all said and done, that I was the first MTC patient my endocrinologist and ENT surgeon had ever seen. I'm not exactly sure why we didn't have that bit of information beforehand, but we didn't. I could have sworn we asked the endocrinologist but he had a great way of closing his eyes, perching his hands and fingers into a prayer like pose and side stepping some of our big questions. I think after that we were being conditioned by these experts not to expect straight answers to our questions. Maybe that's why my surgeon was left off the hook, meaning we may not have asked him how many MTC patients he had in his practice because we didn't expect to be answered or we expected to be ignored. In my defense, it was only after I became a member of the wonderful online ThyCa group that I found all the mistakes I had made by not asking very specific and important questions and holding firm to wait for an answer. But, as I've said we are not ones to dwell in the past. Our mission now is to stay connected with our Meddie friends and arm ourselves with the best information available and move onward and upward. Secondly, our mission is to stay clear of the "running rampant" ideology.

If someone asked me to share a tidbit of guidance to a newly diagnosed Medullary Thyroid Cancer patient, I would say don't let your thoughts or actions run rampant. Proceed slowly, methodically, and armed with as much information as you are able to find and only move forward when you feel comfortable and secure in your decision. And open up and share all of your thoughts and concerns with your Meddie family, they (we) understand what you're going through.

Listen To Those Inner Voices

By Karen Christianson

April 7, 2015, marked my three-year anniversary since being diagnosed with medullary thyroid cancer (MTC). Here's the good news: I cried with delight when my endocrinologist told me that since my numbers hadn't moved much, that the odds were that this disease would not kill me within 10 years. The tears of joy streamed uncontrollably down my face. The only thought I had was that my 11-year-old would have her mom until she was at least 21 years old. We all know losing a parent when one is young defines a part of who you are, and it's not something I wanted for her. As I celebrated the next few weeks with postings on Facebook, email, and the superficial cocktail party, the faces on the people who didn't have cancer or a loved one with cancer looked uncomfortable and at a loss for words. The cancer patients knew exactly where my heart was and immediately and warmly embraced my celebration. That's where I am today.

It all started about five years ago. First, I'm a 5'2", type A, natural redhead who's spent my whole life apologizing for trying to "get life right" because my way is the right and only way of doing things, of course. Confrontation is my way of staying in control of everything, so I embrace it and exercise it frequently. I lost my dad suddenly to liver cancer, and I lost my sister to breast cancer. My sister was diagnosed at stage 4 and valiantly fought for seven years. Those years of her suffering were not at all fun or rewarding. I was very close to the situation.

She died in my arms, which in retrospect has been one of the greatest gifts I've ever received. I tell you this because when I think of cancer, one does not win. Ever. Because of the control freak thing I mentioned earlier, I became a borderline—depending who you talk to—hypochondriac. My fear of cancer was a huge thing in my life. I'm not afraid to die. I'm afraid of the suffering and what it puts your family through.

I'm also quite a spiritual person. I meditate and have a special relationship with a spirit world or guardian angel, whatever you want to name it. Yep, some say I'm crazy and my response is, "If this is crazy, I've never been happier."

In my dreams or times of thought I kept choking, or had trouble talking. Every conscious thought had to do with my throat. Since I was rounding the corner to turning 50, I was interpreting it as "Shut up and listen for once." So I tried listening classes. Tried to be sensitive. The dreams and voices and thoughts got louder and louder, so I asked my GP to check my throat. After I begged him to give me an ultrasound of my neck, we found the lump. Everyone said lumps on your thyroid are extremely common and nothing to worry about. After a needle biopsy proved it was benign, I was told to forget about it. Not so easy for the control freak who's afraid of cancer, but I tried.

The symptoms started about a year later. Diarrhea every single morning. Not enough to wreck my day, but it was there every day. I became quite a chemist trying to figure out why. I blamed it on the magnesium and turmeric I was taking to help sleep and manage inflammation. It didn't work. The sweating was also something else. There would be seemingly a gallon of sweat all at once, dripping and happening at all times during the day. I learned it is called flushing. The lethargy was also weird for me. I had always been a freak about working out, and yep, I would overdo it and love it. Endorphins are my Prozac. But now, I couldn't make it through a day without a nap.

Guess what the Medical Community said? Hormones. For any girl over 40 the answer is typically hormones. This really pisses me off because I think it happens a lot. The funny thing is, the blood work at my physical did not agree with the Medical Community, but they didn't care. It was still hormones. Ugh.

Then something cool happened. I sat at a bar with a neighbor friend who's a doctor. One of the sweating episodes was happening and I asked her if she wanted to see a "live" hot flash happening. "Watch me," I said. As the water started to drip she made one comment: "I don't think that's a hot flash. Your neck isn't red at all."

I got on the Internet and started the self-diagnosis. I begged my friend, who's an ENT, to take another look at my thyroid. It was a Sunday afternoon, but he opened his office. My husband and he fumbled to turn on the ultrasound machine. I've had five babies, so I could do it blindfolded. Anyway, after comparison he said, "Well, it hasn't grown, but it's now follicular." I've stared at enough of my sister's x-rays to know we don't like the word or the looks of a follicular tumor.

Another needle biopsy indicates it's benign. "No need to worry," the Medical Community said. WRONG ANSWER, I thought. I couldn't do it.

After about a week my ENT friend called and said, "I know you're a worrier. Let's take out half of your thyroid. You'll have the other half, so things will be easy. I've done it thousands of times. It's not a big deal."

The surprise was I immediately said, "Yes, let's do it." Two weeks later his friend operated on me, taking out the right side of my thyroid. I was criticized by many people for having this surgery. They called it "unnecessary" and remarked, "This is what's wrong with the health care system." The frozen biopsy still said benign. The only comment the surgeon said afterward was, "I didn't like the way it felt." They sent my cells off to the laboratory. They were supposed to get back to me within two to three days. After three days, I freaked. My friend called and said the UW lab couldn't call it and had it sent to Mayo. He said, "Don't take any aspirin or ibuprofen, just in case"

IN CASE WHAT? Twenty-four hours later I was in the ER with a migraine, puking and having what I would consider a nervous breakdown. My dear friend walked into the ER and told me I had been diagnosed with MTC. I responded, "Yay, if this is cancer, then thyroid cancer is the best one to get, right?"

No, it's the worst freaking one to get.

It's a killer. It's a cut-out disease. You just keep getting tumors cut out because they don't respond to chemo or radiation. Yuck.

One of my many collapsing-on-the-floor moments was talking about the removal of thyroid and total neck dissection that someone described to me over the phone. Two weeks later I got the other side of my thyroid taken out. The surgeon didn't do the neck dissection. He made the call. He thought it was encapsulated and felt all my glands and nodules, and honestly just made the call. It's not standard, but I trust this guy.

Then I had the meeting with my endocrinologist that was burned into my memory. She started saying things like survival rate, saying you have cancer, saying scans, x-rays, blood work every three months. I went numb. I saw her lips moving, but nothing registered. Thank God my husband was there. I was numb, absolutely numb.

The next week of tests and scans honestly were the worst. My stress level was off the charts. I did have some moments I will cherish. I was home and literally fell on the floor, crying. My daughter came home from high school. She picked me up in her arms and carried me to my bed. She talked to me. She loved me. She cared for me. My teenage son hugged me in bed without a word. I apologized to my kids because I'm the one who's supposed to care for them. They didn't have to say words. They just helped me and loved me. I thought to myself, "If this is what I'm on earth to do, then I'm not doing too badly. These are good kids." I've since learned that all five kids dealt with my cancer diagnoses differently, but all would say it was a monumental event in their life.

A scan was performed to show us where the cancer had spread. We waited and waited. It was a Friday afternoon, and my husband had not been to work in two weeks. We were alone in the house. The scan came back clear. The blood work came back clear. We renamed that day Fantastic Friday! I may have gotten to it early. Now that collapse onto the floor with my husband was also worth remembering. I never really could picture or describe JOY until that moment. It was very tangible. We got it early, but don't be too excited, because this slow-growing disease does not have a cure and does not respond to chemotherapy or radiation, so hold that thought.

Medullary thyroid cancer is a patient disease. We watch it. We get blood work every three months and watch a few very specific markers. Calcitonin and CEA are the two major ones. Calcitonin seems to be the marker that says yes or no to this disease. I've asked why we can't test everyone with a lump for calcitonin and I've been told it's too expensive. Great. A blood test is too expensive to save a life. Bull crap on that. I've been rallying to change this fact.

I've also been blown away at how the blood work is handled. Each time I have to tell them that I will fast for the test and I have to tell them to have the blood frozen right away. God forbid if I was shy and didn't speak up for myself.

So it's been three years of blood work and a rewind on how to live. Yep, cancer is the great control-alt-delete in life. You need to chill out a bit and not take things too seriously, and yep, I'm grateful in a way. If anyone's reading this who doesn't have cancer, please remember a few things. Please don't say, 'Oh good, thyroid cancer is the best cancer to get." It sucks no matter which kind you have, and MTC is not the more common and treatable thyroid cancer. You cannot put the level of pain and stress on a human being when they hear their doctor say, "You have cancer," no matter what kind it is. The stress before and during and waiting for results from the testing is outrageous. I've bought and gone to every workshop about stress and mindfulness, but that waiting for results hurts no matter what.

The Facebook listserv I joined on my cancer, MTC, is an example of human kindness and love. This is a group of people who have instant equanimity. We have one thing in common: We suffer with this disease. Nothing else matters to these people. They don't care what color you are, or where you're from. They don't care what religion you are. Hey, they don't even care how much money you make. They love and support everyone equally. It's really remarkable. It's hopeful.

The support from my family and close friends disappoints me. My extended family thinks my cancer is over and doesn't even ask me about my health. My friends think the page has turned on another one of Karen's drama stories. Nope, it's an everyday thing. Every stomachache, bout of diarrhea, or sweat becomes a worry to me. Yes, my cancer prognosis looks good right now. I'm lucky for many things in life. I'm grateful for many, many more. I do, however, stay close to my listserv family who suffer daily from this nasty disease and who lose their lives. It's real, and it's painful.

So, that's the story. Get your thyroid checked regularly. Thyroid cancer is the number one fastest growing cancer. No wonder, with our environment, so be aware. If you have a lump, get the right blood work done ASAP. Be a brash, aggressive advocate for your own health. "Hormones" is not always the answer to the health concern of every woman's over 40. Trust your inner voice! "Live life with an open heart and open mind" is my new motto. Wish me luck. I just turned 50. Here comes menopause!

Take It Day By Day

By Terri Passanesi

My name is Terri Passanesi. I have been married to my amazing husband, Rick for 35 years. I am a mother of three kids, and the proud grandma of five little angles. I am a full time realtor in New York and New Jersey.

In the fall of 2001, I began to notice my hair was thinning a little. I also found a lump in the center of my neck. I ignored the lump at first, as so many of us do, being busy taking care of our families, working, and going along with our busy schedules. When I finally went to the doctor, he sent me for a thyroid uptake to see if there was a problem with my thyroid. This test showed everything to be ok with my thyroid, so he told me to leave it alone.

A year later during a routine checkup, I asked him if I should be concerned that this has not gone away. That was about a year after I felt it. He suggested that I see an endocrinologist, and recommended one in Staten Island, where I live. During the exam with this endo, he gave me a glass of water and felt my neck. He said it was nothing and to go home and take some aspirin. Needless to say, I never went back to him.

In the beginning of 2003, I went back to my primary care doctor and told him that I was very concerned that this lump was still there, and that it had become annoying. He told me to see a surgeon. He still believed that it was nothing too serious, but if I felt better removing it, then that is what I should do. I went to see a very good general surgeon who came highly recommended to me. He thought that even if it was benign, if it made me uncomfortable it should be removed. He said that he would only take the right lobe, where the lump was. The left lobe would produce enough hormone that I would probably not need any medication.

I went for surgery in July 2003. When it was over, Dr. Steinbruck told my husband that he believed that the tumor was cancerous. The pathology proved it to be Medullary Thyroid Cancer. He suggested that I see Dr. Tuttle in Memorial Sloan Kettering. I did not want to go there!! That was a cancer hospital and I was not ready to admit that I had cancer. I scheduled my second surgery with Dr. Steinbruck in September 2003. He insisted that if I didn't want to see Dr. Tuttle, I should at least see a skilled endocrinologist, like Dr. Blum at NYU.

When I went to see him, he took one look at my file and said "Medullary Thyroid Cancer? I don't treat that." Up to that point I had not cried about the whole cancer thing. But when this doctor, a man who is highly regarded in his field, refused to treat me, I lost it. I could not imagine what was growing inside of me that was so horrible that I could not be treated. I left his office crying. My husband, Rick, did not leave with me. He stayed and insisted that if he was not going to help me then he should find someone who can. Like Dr. Stienbruck, Dr. Blum said that the best place for me was MSKCC with Dr. Tuttle. Rick stayed in his office until he got an appointment to see Dr. Tuttle.

I have been under his care since. In 2008 my CEA and my calcitonin had increased enough so that I had to have a modified radical right neck dissection, and this was done at MSKCC by Dr. Shaha. I know that there is another surgery in my near future, but as of last scans and tests, it won't be this year.

I know I am in good hands now. I have a doctor who sees many MTC patients each week. I had to come to grips with going to a cancer center. Everything about cancer was very overwhelming at first. This type of cancer, the "good" kind, is like waiting for the other shoe to drop. You never know when it will be coming back again, and whether it will stay only in my neck, or travel to other organs, as has happened to too many of my meddie friends. All we can do it take it day by day.

My Body's Betrayal

By Mahaut de la Mare

When I was first diagnosed with MTC (Medullary Thyroid Cancer) by my ENT, I was horrified! I really only heard the word "cancer". My own body had betrayed me, and two years before, cancer had claimed my daddy. I watched my once healthy daddy shrink to an elderly person. He was no longer able to eat. His wife was taking him to MUSC for an operation where they would try to give him more time by cleaning out some of the tumors in his neck. They opened one side first, and from what they saw, they knew it would make no difference. They were going to send him home on Hospice, but the cancer couldn't even let us have that. The day after daddy awoke, he had a massive heart attack.

My grandmother said he told her "Happy Birthday", then she heard the phone drop, a lot of people in the room with him….then someone hung the phone up. My grandmother never celebrated her birthday again. After she died, my grandfather was diagnosed with colon cancer. Thankfully it was caught early, and my grandfather just celebrated his 90th birthday. So, cancer is no stranger to my family, I had just hoped it was done with us. I was wrong, very wrong.

In June of 2012, I went to my ENT for a lump in my mouth. He did a thorough head and neck exam. While palpating my thyroid, he said "Uh-oh, you have a nodule on your left and right thyroid." I went numb. All I could think about was my daddy, what he went through before he died. Then came the flurry of tests, a needle aspiration, a radioactive test that for the very first time made me a claustrophobic and I still suffer from it. After all the tests came back inconclusive, my doctor said it needed to come out. So out it went. And as it left, it pulled me into early menopause, hot/cold sensations within minutes, and a lot of small but torturous inconveniences.

After surgery, he told me, not only did I have MTC but also Papillary. Luckily they got out all the Papillary, but the lymph nodes they harvested showed that the MTC was microscopically making its way through my body. I can no longer donate my blood, even though it's the rarest type and is needed. I can no longer donate any organs or skin, eyes and such. My body is MTC's playground, anytime, anywhere a tumor (or tumors) finds a good place to latch on.

What if it decides to enter my brain? What parts of "who I am" would have to be sacrificed to keep me alive (providing, of course that they can be operated on). Would I know myself? My children? Mother, sisters? My beloved husband?

It took me many months to stop thinking what *might happen* because it would send me into a panic attack. I would (and sometimes still do) research this rare disease. I have a psychiatrist and a psychologist, and I have an antidepressant and anti-anxiety meds that help. I hope to wean off of them someday.

The saving grace for me was finding out, from testing the actual tumor, that I was a sporadic. That means I couldn't have passed it to my children. And even though they are grown men, I'd like to stay around and see what they will do with their lives. My CEA and Calcitonin levels are staying low, so no tumors yet.

The meddie family on Fb is a Godsend. There is so much knowledge there, and if needed, we can speak about our fears; we can break out the anxiety train knowing we aren't being judged. We are there for each other, and we miss those who have gone before us.

I am still a newbie, still learning, and in a way, still in shock. When it's time to check my blood levels and get scans, I get tense, anxious, and scared until I get the results. Then, I try to push my fears to the back of my mind, and get back to living.

What Cause Would Be Taking Up My Time?

By Kathryn Brubaker Wall

Let me talk about being diagnosed with MTC. I was 35, married, a stay-at-home mom and a hypochondriac. I had two small daughters, ages five and three. Suspecting I had strep throat, I went to my physician assistant, and he noticed a lump on my thyroid. At the time I had no idea what a thyroid did, or where it was located. Everyone kept assuring me it was only a five percent chance it was thyroid cancer, so I thought my chances were good. Turns out I'd won the rare disease lottery.

I was referred to a high volume thyroid surgeon (of course, I didn't know that was important). But I refused to have a Fine Needle Biopsy because I was terrified of needles and the idea of surgery was more appealing to me. (Really? A 35-year-old? You were a real baby!)

This is what I was told over and over again by the doctors and friends who were in the medical field: "Hey, you don't really need a thyroid. You can take a pill each day instead. And even if it is thyroid cancer, don't worry. That's the good cancer. If you have to get cancer, that's the kind you want."

So, I had my thyroidectomy in August 1999, and it turned out I had Medullary Thyroid Cancer, a rare cancer. I immediately got on the Internet and was horrified. I was going to die, or at the very least need multiple surgeries. My anxiety went out the roof. Convinced that I was going to die, I started throwing out stuff I didn't want the church ladies finding when they came to help my husband and small children after I was gone.

My oldest daughter started kindergarten right after my thyroidectomy, which was another huge life shock for me. My husband and I had been married for 11 years when I was diagnosed with MTC. Considering myself a feminist, I had not changed my name when I got married. It caused a fair amount of confusion in my life, but I put up with it because I thought it was important. After I was diagnosed with MTC, I changed my name. That's why for several years I transitioned between using my maiden and married name. My thinking was twofold: First, I didn't want things to be awkward for my daughter in school having an involved mom with a different last name. Second, I figured I was going to die and I wanted my last name to be listed as my married name. (And let me tell you, Wall is a whole lot easier to spell than Brubaker.)

My husband and I had quite a bit of struggle dealing with my cancer diagnosis. I was eager to find out as much as possible, even the bad and negative things that kept me crazy. He found this overwhelming and kept telling me I needed to stop spending so much time on the Internet and dwelling on things.

Where was I spending so much of my time? On the ThyCa Medullary email support group. The group had started in May of that year and I joined it in August 1999. The first person I heard from was Vera, who was the moderator of the group at the time. I will never forget her first email in response to my newbie message of help, I'm newly diagnosed. "I'm Vera and I have mets to the lungs, mets to the liver, have had xx number of surgeries, etc. "I remember feeling like I'd been punched in the gut. I had to go lie down for a while and try to quell the terror.

The "Meddies" told me it was important to go to a specialist. I was my local surgeon's first MTC case. In response to my questions from the online MTC group he told me, "Don't believe anything you read on the Internet." I asked him a few other questions that he didn't like. He ordered an MIBG scan for me at Duke. According to the MTC group, this was an outdated test in 1999, and it showed my doctors' inexperience. My surgeon didn't appreciate the opinion of people on the Internet. I wasn't sure who to believe and what to do.

My surgeon had told me my central lymph nodes had "looked fine," so he didn't remove them. He ordered a calcitonin. (This experience was a disaster and I could write another whole story about my awful experiences over 15 years in getting calcitonin pulled.) It came back at 4000. He said he was certain it was lab error, because he thought it might be around 200. He ordered a second calcitonin, and it was 4100. That was it. I decided to deal with his wrath and seek a second opinion. He wasn't very pleased, and I didn't return to see him again.

This turned out to be very bad, because the surgeon was the one who had prescribed my Synthroid. I was never referred to an endocrinologist or reminded that I should be. I never had my TSH tested after my thyroidectomy. I felt kind of like crap, but I assumed that was because I was terrified. I had no understanding of TSH and that I should have been getting blood tests to check my levels. Plus, I was still freaked out about getting labs done, so it never entered my mind. My original surgery was in August 1999. My TSH was tested for the first time in March 2000, after my neck dissection. My TSH was 36. Normal is between .5 and 3.30. There was a reason why I thought I was losing my mind and was having suicidal thoughts!

The high calcitonin made it apparent I needed a more thorough neck surgery. I went to Duke University, not far from my home in Raleigh. At the time they didn't have a surgeon who would perform this surgery and they made a formal referral to Dr. Jeff Moley in St. Louis, Missouri. I contacted Mary DeBennedetti in Dr. Moley's office and she was an angel to work with. They were quite used to having out-of-town/state/country medullary patients fly in for surgery. They had the process down. We flew in on Thursday morning and met Dr. Moley Thursday afternoon. We checked into the hospital early Friday morning for pre-op tests and had surgery all day Friday. On Sunday I was discharged to a hotel. Monday morning I got checked and had a calcium-stimulated calcitonin test. Monday afternoon I flew home. At the time we were under an HMO, and based on letters written on my behalf from my Primary Care Physician and Duke, every bit of the expense was covered, even our hotel room and airfare.

My calcitonin never went back to zero. I am not "cured," although the local endocrinologist to whom I had finally been referred assured me I was. He considered himself an authority on MTC, and I quickly began to understand that doctors are people and they aren't all what they say they are. I kept asking him to set up the RET genetic test for me and he kept stonewalling me. Finally he told me it was not commercially available. It was, but he wouldn't even take the time to bother looking at the papers I'd given him. I was stuck, because at the time his practice was the only endocrinology group in town. I ended up taking my information from Dr. Moley back to my physician assistant and he ordered the test. I got it the next day. That really cemented in my mind that you have to "drive your own bus" (thank you for that jewel, Meddie Friends). You don't have to accept what the doctor says as gospel.

Even though I had been an anxious wreck during the year of my surgeries, I really fell apart around the one-year anniversary of my neck dissection. A lot had to do with the horrible rollercoaster of TSH and the effect it had on my body. But more had to do with the devastating diagnosis of cancer, my tendency to hypochondria and feeling so out of control. My saving grace was the medullary email group, going to ThyCa conferences and my Stephen Minister at church. Having someone to talk to was so important. I found I couldn't share freely with my family and friends. It would upset them too much, or they would just try to shut me down. "You worry too much. You shouldn't read all that stuff on the Internet." Even my local endocrinologist told me he didn't understand why I would want to be involved with ThyCa because I was "cured" and didn't I want to move on with my life? (I see a different endocrinologist these days.)

ThyCa evolved into a big part of my life, and my volunteer activities have expanded over the years. I went to conferences in 2000 and

2001. I started the local Raleigh thyroid cancer support group in 2005 and I'm still facilitating the group today. I kept coming back to ThyCa Conferences, and in time, I started facilitating some round tables. It became an expected thing that "Mom's conference" was every fall, and I always tried to go. In 2010, I was asked to join the board of directors of ThyCa, and I try very hard to represent the Medullary voice. It's not very hard, because Gary Bloom, our executive director, is very aware of the medullary community and he has always made a point of looking out for our concerns. In 2011, Gary asked me to help fill in with a program need, helping new people start ThyCa Support Groups in their own communities. When I said yes, I only intended to do it short term. But I found that I really enjoyed working with the facilitators, who are some of ThyCa's most dedicated volunteers. I just kept meeting more and more great people. It's been a wonderful experience, and due to my increased work schedule and the increase in new groups, I'm mainly helping with existing groups now. My most recent ThyCa involvement is working on the social media team and helping with Facebook.

Like I said at the very beginning of this, if I had never had thyroid cancer, what cause would be taking up so much of my time? I just don't know. But I wouldn't change a thing.

When You Get A Second Cancer

By Kathryn Brubaker Wall

I've been giving some thought to what my life would look like if I had never had a cancer diagnosis 16 years ago. This is really hard to imagine, because so much of my time and so many of my friends are thyroid cancer survivors. Some of the most rewarding and fulfilling parts of my life right now are wrapped around thyroid cancer support. So after I consider everything, I don't regret getting cancer and going through this. I would not trade the good that came from the bad. It definitely has helped shape me into the person I am today.

I'll get back to my original diagnosis in a little bit, but I want to talk about something that terrifies a lot of women, especially those who have had thyroid cancer. Two years ago I was diagnosed with breast cancer. I started having mammograms around age 40, but they had always been negative and I got lazy and skipped a couple of years before I realized it. In early 2013 I got around to having one done, since I have a family history of breast cancer. When I got a phone call to come in for a diagnostic mammogram after my regular one, I kind of knew immediately that it probably was cancer. In the weeks before this diagnosis I had been having severe anxiety attacks related to my work (so I thought) and had just started seeing a counselor in the week before the breast cancer diagnosis. This was eerily like my medullary diagnosis. I had experienced extreme anxiety attacks and had sought out counseling the year up to my diagnosis. In retrospect you could either say it was a coincidence, or perhaps my sixth sense was telling me something was about to happen.

I've immersed myself in the cancer support world for many years, attended ThyCa conferences and spoken with top physicians. But I had forgotten how many misconceptions are out there about cancer. People say stupid stuff. I got asked some of the strangest questions. A lot of people assumed because I said I had breast cancer, I was apparently going to die.

I hated having to deal with cancer angst again. You know what I'm talking about. People asking me, "How are you?" and knowing I was the subject of concern and pity. (That poor Kathryn. Two cancers!) Even though I was exasperated at having to go through this again, I did have the benefit of perspective this time around. I have a relative who chose not to tell her elderly father that she had cancer and I had judged her severely for withholding that information. This time around I could totally see her point of view and was much more understanding. I hated telling everyone. Having to call my parents and tell our children was really difficult. I just didn't want to worry anyone.

The breast cancer was caught pretty early and I didn't have any lymph node involvement. I chose to do a lumpectomy, which was done outpatient. After the procedure and before I went home, the Nurse Navigator arrived in my hospital room with a hot pink bag. Inside was a handmade pillow (made by breast cancer survivors), a bunch of stuff I don't remember, and a two-sided handout. The handout had a list of names and phone numbers. These were the people I could call for help: the Nurse Navigator, nutritionist, massage therapist, support group, numbers for the oncology department, radiation oncology department, genetic counselor, etc. Wow. With MTC I had been on my own in finding any of those things. But that pink bag really bothered me. I wasn't sure I wanted to be identified as a breast cancer survivor. The over-commercialization of breast cancer awareness turns me off. Now I had to decide how this was going to change me and how it would change my identity.

For me, breast cancer was more of an annoyance than a trauma, unlike my original MTC diagnosis. I was aggravated that I had to deal with it. I had to add many new doctors, and it was very expensive. Even with "good" insurance, we spent almost $20,000 out of pocket. After some genetic tumor testing, we agreed that chemotherapy wasn't necessary, and after the lumpectomy I ended up doing six weeks of external beam radiation. One of the first days I took a photo of the machine and posted it on Facebook. In my mind, I was sharing the room and how it looked for my mom, my husband and my older daughters. "Look how cool this is" I wanted to show. By the time I got home, my Facebook was flooded with "Oh, you poor thing" type of commentary, and I have to say it bothered me. I felt like I was trolling for sympathy, or people thought I was scared by this enormous machine.

I've really found that your reaction to my cancer is more about you than it is me.

The Squirrelly Kind Of Cancer

By Tami Weaver

Cancer is something that affects every family in some way, either directly or indirectly. You always think, "This won't happen in my family or to me." Cancer doesn't care. If it wants to come into your life, it will. It doesn't care if you're in the best shape or the worst shape, if you're male or female, young or old, married or single. It can get you, whether you want it to, or not.

I had never heard of thyroid cancer, let alone Medullary Thyroid Cancer (MTC). Imagine my surprise when I found out I had the "squirrelly" kind. It was after surgery, 33 external beam radiation treatments and my doctors not seeming to agree, that I started to research MTC. It's all very overwhelming. I've since transferred to a Center of Excellence and am on the wait and see program. This seems to be a current trend among Meddies.

People have often commented, "I don't know how you do it." Granted, there are good days and bad days, but life goes on, one day at a time. It's hard to accept when a fellow Meddie passes away. You panic over every ache and pain. Your pinky toe starts to hurt, and you think, "Oh my, the cancer has spread to my toe!" That's why I'm on prescription "happy pills." Not sure they always work. "It is what it is" has become my motto.

You often wonder, why me? We don't know. I seem to be the "go-to" thyroid expert at work. I don't always have the answer, but I try. I tell everyone to check their necks.

Hopefully, with the publication of our Meddie Memoirs, we can raise more awareness to this "squirrelly" kind of cancer.

It is what it is.

The Diagnosis

By Sue Evert

I guess you could say my journey began in April 2009, when my daughter started working at a gynecologist's office; she made an appointment for me, knowing that I had not been to one in years. I had the routine checkup and a mammogram, which came back with questionable findings meaning I would need to have another one done. At that second appointment, I never expected that a doctor and nurse would pull me into a room to talk to me about what they saw, yet that's what happened. They were both very serious and told me I needed to get to a specialist as soon as possible and schedule a breast biopsy, and gave me a folder with a whole bunch of articles about breast cancer. I don't even remember the drive home I just remember thinking are you kidding me? I've done the standard breast exams I've never felt anything. Ok, maybe I wasn't great about going to doctors as I've never had any luck with them helping me with various other issues over the past 5+ years. Anyway, needless to say, I called and made an appointment with a well-known breast cancer surgeon in our area and scheduled an appointment to discuss the biopsy procedure. It was during that appointment that the Doctor pointed out the lump in my neck and started asking me questions about it. I am pretty sure I was like, "Oh, that's just my Adam's Apple or something, I've had it for a long time and I just assumed it was a part of me". No one had ever asked me about it. I didn't know if the size was changing I just knew it was there. I don't think I even knew what a thyroid was or that I even had one (and yes I'm very serious about that). Within the next couple of weeks I was getting two biopsies done.

In the meantime, I began researching all I could about breast cancer and thyroid cancer while my family told me to stop. In my heart I knew one of them (if not both) were going to end up coming back as a cancer. Not the best attitude to have but just being truthful. I keep coming across article after article saying that Thyroid Cancer is a good cancer, it's treatable & curable so hey, at that point I was thinking, "Well, if these are my two options then I hope it's the good curable one." All the while thinking, "How is there such a thing as a good cancer?"

My breast biopsy came back first and it was benign, whew! one down, one to go. After that I had the follow up appointment in regards to my thyroid nodule biopsy, and, "Well, there's a little problem and we can't really say right now, but we sent everything to Duke University to have them look at it and I'll get back to you". Now I really started researching thyroid cancers and I found out about the 4 different types you can get. As I was reading about the different types I came across the very little description of Medullary Thyroid Cancer (MTC as we now call it) and my heart sunk as I knew this was what I had, in fact, there was no doubt in my mind that I had this.

You see, I have and continue to have each and every side effect listed with MTC. I can't even tell you how many specialists I saw because of the uncontrollable diarrhea I have suffered with for the past 5-7 years, no one was ever able to tell me why I had so many issues, test after test kept just coming back saying it's IBS, or lactose intolerance, too much stress, you don't eat right, of course you're tired, you are not getting enough nourishment. And all the time my TSH has always been normal, and because MTC is rare, the little calcitonin test that would have diagnosed me a lot sooner, was never done.

I was officially diagnosed with MTC the week of my 42nd birthday, June of 2009. When I walked into that follow up appointment my ENT still wasn't sure how to tell me I had this disease. A disease he personally has never seen or treated, and I finally blurted it out to him, "I know it's Medullary Thyroid Cancer, right"? I then told him of my research and that I had every side effect listed for MTC.

I didn't know about centers of excellence, and how important getting the correct surgery was, but my ENT did and he wanted to refer me to one of them, but I chose to stay with him. He already had been talking to a friend and surgeon at University of Pennsylvania. He recommended I go there, but he said he thought he could do the surgery, too, and the decision was up to me. All I knew was that I liked this doctor, I was comfortable with him, and I was comfortable that he was working with the surgeon from Penn, so I decided on the guy who was close to my home and my family. I look back on all of this now as a complete blur, but I was a newbie. I had no idea whatsoever what I was getting myself into. I was scared as all hell, everything I'm reading is that only 3%-5% of the population get this, and by the time that person is diagnosed it's pretty late for them and the overall chance of long term survival is well, NULL. I am literally putting my life in his hands and even today almost 6 years later I do not regret that decision at all, in fact because of this man's inexperience, he did more tests than they would have normally done, and when the cancer had spread to my liver within 3 months of surgery, I would not have had the same treatment options I ended up with.

Now comes the worst part, how do you tell your family, your loved ones, this type of news? How to I pretend that I'm not scared to death, that this is nothing. I'm strong. I can do it. I pull up my big girl panties, pretend that I am not sick, I'm not scared, and that we will beat this together. I explain how rare it is and there doesn't seem to be a cure for it, so basically I have this huge surgery and then we wait and see what happens next. I try to not cry too much as I don't want them to be scared too. What a mess, how/why did this happen to me? Why, when I was going through both possible situations, breast cancer and thyroid cancer, did I think I was getting off easy if I ended up with thyroid cancer? I think sometimes it's Karma for me even thinking that any cancer was good. And now I fully got to learn that no cancer is easy, and that it's a damn shame that any cancer is perceived this way. If our stories change anything, it's my hope that people will learn something that I didn't know myself until I got cancer: there is NO such thing as a Good cancer, no one gets a break. Being told you have cancer is one of worst experiences you can ever have. Period.

With my family and friends rallying around me, and boy do I mean rally (the doctors and nurses said they had never before seen so many loved ones and such a supportive gathering in the waiting room), I had my 8-hour surgery (2 days before our 23rd wedding anniversary) and everything went smoothly. I healed well, the pain was tolerable, the scar a lot better than I imagined. I was able to come home 3 days later to await the results of my pathology report. Those reports came back not clear, not within normal margins and it's determined I am stage 4b. Now, the man I had trusted completely has no other option but to refer me to those specialists at University of Pennsylvania for further surgeries or other options. I started to recover while still trying to wrap my head around all that had happened those 3 months. But I stayed strong, trying not to dwell on what lay ahead. I went back to work on a part time basis. I had my first appointment with the new specialist, who went over my reports and determined that I needed to get another biopsy and possibly another surgery, that things were more difficult than they first thought. I was also sent for more tests (MRI's, CT scans) and would also have to meet with the surgeon after those specialists had a meeting with the tumor review board. My head was spinning. Tumor Review Board? What the hell does that mean??? I am beyond scared, but continue to try and just focus on my family, my job and my life. I went to the next appointment to meet the surgeon and found out what was decided that I should do. The guy basically said, "NOTHING". We left that meeting utterly confused and thinking, "If this guy is an expert, man I'd hate to see what a non-expert was". The following day while I was at work, I got a phone call from the endocrinologist from U of Penn and she began to inform me over the phone that the reason the surgeon wasn't informative was because my cancer had already metastasized into my liver, and that surgery was no longer a viable option. I now needed to go to the hospital that did the surgery, pick up my tissues and the reports and to get back to Penn immediately (the next day) to meet with an oncologist to discuss whatever options I may have left. Did you notice that I said, "ON THE PHONE"???? Yes, I was told via telephone, by a so called professional doctor that my cancer had spread to my liver. That yes, it means we don't really have any other options for you and that yes you need to prepare yourself for your impending death. And what can I do? I started screaming and crying. I fall into a heap on the floor by my desk, in front of numerous co-workers and completely lost my mind. My boss, who thankfully sits right next to me and who also happens to be one of my best friends, grabbed me off the floor, pulled me into a conference room, and picked up her phone to call my husband. The entire floor of our office building heard it all, saw it all, and to this day, they have a hard time looking me in the eye (and I know they do, too). They got to see first-hand, how utterly devastated a person is when they are told they are going to die. I think all of them experienced their lives flashing before their eyes. To this day, I still cannot believe that a doctor would tell a person this type of news over the phone, and because I was in shock, and everything was a complete whirlwind after that, I never complained to the hospital board about this experience. I know I should have even though it doesn't take away the shame for me, it might have helped her to learn not to do this to another person. That's the beginning of my journey…

Living With MTC

By Sue Evert

In June of 2004, Tim McGraw released a song called "Live Like You Were Dying" that touched me in ways I never expected. I broke down in tears the first time I heard it, as it had so much meaning. And that was 5 years before I became the person in that song! The song begins like this, "I was in my early 40's with a lot of life before me, when I got the news that stopped me on a dime."

In June of 2009 the week of my 42nd birthday, I was officially diagnosed with a rare form of thyroid cancer (Medullary Thyroid cancer – MTC as we call it). I was informed that this type of cancer is rare, has no cure, with very few treatment options. "How does it hit'cha when you get that kind of news?" It's mind-blowing, you can't breathe, you want to run away and hide, you want to wake up from this horrible dream and pray that it was just a nightmare and that your world has not really turned upside down. But in all reality, those are not options when in fact you have to do the complete opposite. You try to let it sink in and then you try to face the reality of your own immortality and how in the hell do you tell your family this dreadful news? I have a husband that I've been with for over 20 years. I have a 21 year old daughter, a brand new 6 month old grandson, my mom, my dad, my sister and my brother who are not only my siblings are my very best friends. I had nieces, nephews, other family, and close friends that are the family of my heart. I can't possibly tell them that this it, that I have 4-5 years before this cancer kills me. How can I leave them? I haven't seen my daughter get married; my grandson doesn't even know who I am yet. I want to celebrate my silver wedding anniversary, why is this happening to me, to us?

Ok, buck up, girl. Be strong, you can't let anyone know how scared you are, because if you lose it then so will they, and you're the glue that keeps everyone together. So stand up, brush yourself off and fight! fight! with every breath you have left. It's time to really start living your life, and now you can do it with your eyes and heart wide open.

In October of 2009, just 3 short months after being diagnosed, I was informed that my cancer had spread to my liver. That it was scattered throughout my entire liver, and I had very limited options. Thankfully I was close to University of Pennsylvania and an oncologist there was just starting a clinical trial drug for MTC. Thankfully I had an inexperienced doctor when I was first diagnosed and he ran more tests than he needed. This allowed me to prove how aggressive my cancer was, otherwise I would not have been approved for the trial. You had to show progression within a 6-month time frame, the initial doctor had an MRI of my abdomen done in June, which showed no liver lesions, yet when reimaged in October of that same year, I had them scattered throughout my liver. So this now enabled me to get into the trial for XL184. This drug is now one of two FDA-approved treatment options for MTC and it is working to keep my cancer levels stable. The drug is now at more tolerable dosage level than when we started. I started at 300 mgs, which was toxic for me, and I imagine it's toxic for everyone on it. I immediately started with hand, foot and mouth sores. Sores so bad in my mouth and throat I could not even swallow, let alone eat. The diarrhea that is already a side effect of the cancer and something that you think can't possibly get worse, became so bad that I practically lived in the bathroom. The side effects were so severe, but the drug was working and keeping my cancer from growing. Because of those results my doctor started playing around with the rules, which then allowed me to reduce the dosage and take some breaks from treatment. Because of those breaks, I was able to endure the medicine for an almost unheard of 16 months, when I finally made the decision to stop treatment. It was killing me quicker than the cancer, and I knew then, exactly what quality of life over quantity meant, and with my eyes wide open, I chose quality.

Telling my family I was stopping was probably the second hardest thing I've ever had to do. When I got to 80 lbs., I knew that was the day I was going to stop the treatment, and that day happened in June of 2011, actually on my mom's birthday. But we didn't tell my family until later as we didn't want to ruin her day. I didn't debate it with them, as the decision was not open for discussion. The only thing I asked was that they love me and support my decision. While it broke their hearts to agree, they supported me whole-heartedly. At the time I made the decision to stop treatment, there were no other options available and I basically went on palliative care with my oncologist. I had my first appointment 3 months later, and my scans showed that in just that short time frame, my liver was now encased with lesions (they stopped counting at 30). She shared the news that another drug had just been approved for MTC patients (Caprelsa) and she wanted me to start immediately. I really didn't think I had it in me to do another round of treatment because the first one was so horrendous. She explained that this one was showing a lot of promise and that treatment side effects had been mild, and that because this was an approved drug, I was not restricted to dosage levels. If I couldn't tolerate it, we would adjust it. Before deciding I had to ask, "If I do nothing, what am I looking at"? She said at best guess 6 months to a year based on how quickly the cancer was growing. I looked at my husband, thought of my family, and knew that 6 months wasn't enough time to do what I still wanted to do. In 6 months my grandson still would not have his own memories of me, and that thought alone made me say yes, but I'll do it on my own terms. At the first sign of distress, first sign of loss of quality of life again, I will reduce the dose or stop treatment. You see, I had 2 months of good, 2 months of living again, and while it wasn't great, it felt like I could be the person who was living with cancer. I didn't want that feeling to stop.

I am now going into my 3rd year on Caprelsa, and while it hasn't been easy, it has been livable. Overall Caprelsa is keeping my cancer growth stable. I now have tumors in my lungs and spine but they are still within acceptable growth allowances and I still get to enjoy life. I may not be the person I used to be, but I am alive and living my life.

There have been ups and downs. I have at times been on my knees begging for it all to end. And then begging for it not to end, that it's too soon, I am not finished yet, there is still so much left for me to do. And to quote again from my song, "I have gotten to love deeper, gave forgiveness I'd been denying, became the wife I knew I could be, and the friend I'd like to have."

And here I am now, in what will be my 6-year "cancerversary" in June 2015. Thank God I didn't listen to the statistics. Thank God I'm a lot stronger than I ever thought possible. Thank God even more for blessing me with the most amazing family and friends a person could ever ask for. Six years ago everything seemed so bleak. I was mentally preparing my goodbyes, I was updating my will, creating a living will, and I was also writing notes to my daughter for her to read on her wedding day. For my grandson to read when he was old enough, or to one day read by himself. Writing to my parents about how much they had given me, how much I loved them. To my sister and brother for always being by my side. To my husband who has been with me since I was 16 years old, and who has stood beside me day in and day out, never once letting me fall. I was saying my good byes in words that I could only write and not say. I cried when everyone was at work and I was by myself. I cried then because I didn't want them to know how truly sad I was, not to be dying but to be leaving them. I never thought I would have these past 6 years to show them how much they meant to me, to be able to live my life with them as if I were dying, and to cherish each and every single moment of that life.

So what is it like to live your life like you're dying? For me, it's learning the true meaning of love. I have seen and felt so much love that it's hard to explain. At best, all I can say is that I am getting to see and experience something that most people never get to see or feel in their lifetime. I am living as if I am standing outside and watching what my viewing/funeral would be like. I have learned that I really do have the best family and friends ever; they all have been here for me from the beginning. From day one when diagnosed, to the day we cut my hair off. We made it a party, we drank, we laughed, I think we had about 20 people here that day, and there were no tears allowed. Just love and support. They turned around and had my first fundraiser benefit where well over 400 people attended, and almost every guy there shaved his head in my honor. They have been here to hold us up; they have been here mentally, physically, emotionally and even financially. This past year when we got the news that Caprelsa was going to cost us $3,000 a month for at least the first 3 months, they never even hesitated and began fundraising again. The things people do when someone they love is going through something like this is truly amazing and inspiring. It is because of them, that I am continually inspired to fight this disease with everything I have. Each and every time I think I can't do it anymore, they pick me up and show me how I can. That all I need to do is to lean on them and they will get me through the next battle. That together we are cancer strong. I am not alone, together we are all fighting this battle, and together we will stay. While I can never say getting cancer is a blessing, I can say that because of cancer I realize how truly blessed I am. I wish everyone could know what it feels like to live as if you are dying. Those who have stayed beside us during these past 6 years continually tell me how strong I am. I am a fighter, yet I just want them all to know that without all of them, I could not be this strong, I could not fight this as hard. And finally because of them I believe I am a warrior.

One Thing To Be Happy About

By Jo Gorringe

It seems strange to write about the "gifts" of having cancer, but there are some.

I have found out who my real friends are very quickly. The ones who stood by me during the early days of self-pity. Why me? Well, why not me? The ones who were around to drive me to doctor appointments, the lab, and same-day surgeries. The ones who would share their fears and sadness at the idea of losing me. The ones who helped me plan my funeral. The ones who made sure that I ate. The ones who remembered that I needed laughter as well as tears.

I've been able to take part in a clinical trial for a cancer vaccine. An incredible thing. This one is supposed to keep my cancer stable longer. Somewhere along the line they'll use these results, and possibly discover a preventive treatment. That's me, helping to make history! That's absolutely amazing. That an ordinary woman from Columbus, Ohio, could *make history*! An amazing gift.

Finding a new family of other meddies. People who are amazing, interesting, and diverse. It's a joy and a pleasure each time two or more of us get together. We laugh, cry, share information about our common disease, our families, our lives. We find we have much more in common than the beast within us.

Getting acquainted with my own leadership skills. I've always been the one in the corner. No more. If I have a chance to talk about this to anyone at all, I do. We are family with an orphan cancer and most of us continue to work. Because of circumstances, I'm not one of those. That means I have nothing to lose by discussing this beast with complete strangers in airports, the grocery store, my local Starbucks. I'm a lucky woman.

Agreed: This is a short list. But it's not all bad. Am I happy and excited to have cancer? Of course not! Am I foolish enough that I don't make the best of it? Of course not. Every single day, for every single person, there's some one thing to be happy about.

Dancing Through Cancer

By Jo Gorringe

It all started out as a joke. One of the people in our Facebook Meddie Family started teasing me about being a "table dancer." Funny, because I'm a great-grandmother with stage 4 cancer and severe osteoporosis. Then one of the guys in the Family dared me to dance on the table at the annual ThyCa Conference in Denver. On Friday nights at the Conference we have the biggest Meddie Meet-Up of the year. We order pizza, bring in drinks and cookies and celebrate together. It's a lot of fun, and in Denver we were joined by one of our major researchers. There I was, wearing a purple Hawaiian shirt, and I climbed up on the table to dance. Dare answered!

The Meddie Family is an international one, with every religion represented. We also have the usual agnostics, and at least one atheist. The one thing we all share are the stars at night. I refer to those Meddies whom we have lost as "Meddie Stars." It's always painful to lose a family member. I choose to celebrate the lives they've lived by dancing under the stars. I usually cry while I dance, but it's a way to honor those whom we've lost. So Friday night after I danced on the table at our Meet-Up, I dragged everyone out to dance under the Stars, including our wonderful researcher.

Then we decided to take it a step further. At the banquet Saturday night, we auctioned off a table dance and collected over $1,000 for ThyCa research. A silly thing maybe, but a wonderful way to give back.

I chose to dance to the song, "We Are Family" by Sister Sledge. I did have a couple of guys spotting me, but I also raised more than $200 in tips. So our joke turned into a dare, and the dare turned into reality. We ended up rocking out the dance floor! I imagine I'll be "table dancing" at ThyCa Conferences for many years to come. I love my Meddie Family, and I'm no longer joking or being dared. I'm dancing my way through thyroid cancer, and I'm very proud of it!

Keeping It All In Perspective

By Bill Prentice

The world is an imperfect place, and I certainly contribute to that imperfection. Yet life goes on, and for most people, they accept that they'll get up in the morning, go to work, come home, do some chores, go to sleep, and do it all over again tomorrow. That is, until one day a life-changing event happens. Now, the term "life-changing event" may seem self-explanatory, but I can see that your definition and my definition might be different. So let me give you my definition so you can see things in the proper perspective. Life-changing events, to me, are events that - once they occur - change your life irreversibly. There's no going back to the way things were.

To date, approaching age 62, I've had several life-changing events, not all of which were within my control. Sure, getting married, having kids, graduating college, were all life-changing, but, for me, were all planned. The unplanned events are the ones I'm writing about.

My first unplanned life-changing event happened at age 17, when I was critically injured in a house fire. Although the burns healed over the following two years and the lung damage from breathing superheated air improved a bit over a longer time, my life was irreversibly changed. The physical and emotional ashes of that event are with me still. I went into that event a 17-year-old kid and came out a man. That fire defined the adult Bill.

The death of my father ten years after his retirement was another life-changing event. Not only was the family patriarch gone, but suddenly my mother's entire live-in support system disappeared. Thank God for my sister, Mary, for being there to guide and support her through the next 20 years. My father's death totally changed our family dynamics. My mother went from never having made a major decision in her entire married life to being a fairly independent 93-year-old at her death.

Three months prior to the death of my father I faced the sudden death of my first wife, Margaret, from undiagnosed leukemia. She died a week before our son Matthew's fourth birthday. 1984 was not a good year, but I toughed it out as a single parent and learned a lot about being self-sufficient, and even more about myself as a parent.

Fast forward 20 years. A long time of stability that included remarriage, the birth of my daughter, several new houses, a new job, a relocation. You could almost get complacent!

But then the big "C" came knocking! July 2005 I discovered I had *cancer*! Yikes! I always try to find the positive in any situation. I have always said that the house fire was the best thing that ever happened to me, taking me from being a high school kid without much direction to an adult man with driving goals. But Cancer . . . How could I find the positive in that?

It's there, if you just open your eyes to it. *Yes*, it is life-changing. *No*, life will never be the same. You can try to hide from it, live in fear or denial, or just succumb to it. Or you can face it head on. I chose the head-on approach.

Cancer, particularly Medullary Thyroid Cancer (MTC), is no walk in the park. It's a sneaky cancer, one that can sit indolent for years, and then suddenly decide to strike out and kill you. My type, sporadic MTC with RET mutation M918T, is known for being aggressive. In reading the literature about the disease, I discovered that I had every indicator for a poor prognosis. Male, over 50, out of shape, having other health issues, late stage discovery, metastatic tumors in the lymph system, metastatic tumors in distant areas outside the neck, and on and on.

The last decade has been a roller-coaster ride. I've had four major surgeries. The initial total thyroidectomy and bilateral neck dissection, a spinal laminectomy because a metastatic tumor broke a piece of my spine, a bilateral adrenalectomy to "cure" Cushing's Syndrome caused by MTC, and gall bladder removal for the same reason. I've also had numerous external beam radiation sessions trying to slow the spread of metastatic disease and perhaps fifteen other in-patient admissions dealing with side effects of the cancer, the treatment, or other related issues. It's been a busy ten years. In 2014 alone, my insurance was billed $247,000 for my care. Fortunately, I have excellent insurance and my out-of-pocket was minimal.

So when I say it's been a hectic ten years, it's been hectic. But it's also been one of the best decades of my life, particularly in the areas of relationship building, self-growth, and faith. Because of cancer I have been exposed to many, many amazing people. From Bob, the radio DJ who had a brain tumor removed and is now dealing with a rare bone cancer but who has found time to dedicate to the Pediatric Brain Tumor Foundation to Becky, now in Florida, who is our illness's survivor community organizer (Watch for her in the next presidential election!), and Jaimie, who turned her life over to God before ever knowing her illness was there, and who leaned on His shoulder to get herself through her treatments *and* the current treatment of her mother for the same hereditary cancer disease! Amazing people, all. And let's not forget Lori, raising a family of three pre-teen and teenage children on the west coast, while dealing with cancer. *I KNOW HOW HARD SINGLE PARENTING IS!* And I was completely healthy throughout my single parenting days. And most recently Rob, a real warrior against his disease, who never gave in or gave up right to the very end. Sadly, he left a mourning wife and two small children behind. Yes, people do die of this disease. 2014 was a particularly bad year, it seemed, and I lost a number of great friends from our Medullary Thyroid Cancer-MTC Facebook group.

Yet life goes on for me, and each day I try to learn and grow. I try to stay positive no matter what is going on. I try to live a faithful life and support others in doing the same, and work harder to show that I love my wife and share my heart with God, all because of Medullary Thyroid Cancer.

So, in keeping things in perspective, thank you, God, for giving me this opportunity to humble myself in front of you, to show you that I am capable of having faith in your direction for my life, and in appreciating the things I have learned from this experience. Your challenges have made me stronger, more faithful, and a better husband, father, and friend.

Remember To Take Care Of Yourself

By Becca

I was first diagnosed with medullary thyroid cancer in December 2000 when I was 21. My daughter was only three at the time. I don't really remember being particularly worried or scared until the night before my first surgery. My mom did all the worrying for me.

Here's my story.

I went to my local community college to get my teeth cleaned by the student dental program there. They told me I had a lump in my neck and needed to get it checked out. I went to my general practitioner, who said it was an infection and he gave me antibiotics. I went through three rounds of antibiotics, but it never went away. So I gave up on the antibiotics.

A few months went by and I got a really bad ear infection. A different doctor gave me a strong antibiotic to clear it up. He said if the knot didn't go away it meant it wasn't an infection.

It was still there after three days, so I went back to him. He sent me to an ENT doctor. I loved her. She was a great doctor and surgeon. I had two fine needle aspirations (FNA) and they both came back inconclusive.

At this point they were leaning towards a diagnosis of papillary thyroid cancer. I went in for my first surgery. It lasted several hours, but then they found out it was MTC, so I had to have a more invasive surgery. They opened up my chest and cut me from ear to ear. A few months later I had radiation.

For several years I was pretty stable. However, my calcitonin and CEA began to go up very gradually, and CT scans revealed signs of progression.

Due to the tumors in my lungs, the doctors decided to start me on TKIs in 2010. They felt that taking out the tumors in my neck wasn't an option, because it might cause me to lose the use of my arm. I started taking a very strong dose of Sutent. It was horrible. The skin rash and mouth sores were awful. My hair turned white. I thought it was falling out, but it was just turning completely white. They lowered my dosage, and it was more tolerable. I was on the medication for about two years, and then the "Big D" started, and I slowly started losing weight.

In 2014 the Sutent stopped working. I was losing weight and the "D" was very bad. They decided to put in a feeding tube to help me get stronger. I went off chemotherapy for a few months and then started taking Caprelsa, with an initial dose of 300mg. However, it was too strong, so they lowered it to 100mg and I did much better with this dosage.

A kind of funny story. I went to the doctor to get my labs done and I'd sit there and worry myself to death about what the numbers might be. I hate needles. I only went there a few times, but the times I'd gone this one guy had done it. This time a lady called me back and said she was going to do my labs. I asked her how long she had been working there and she said, "Oh, I just started." I started crying and wouldn't let her do it. She then told me she was joking and had been doing it for years.

The same guy who started doing my labs 14 or so years ago is still doing my labs to this day. The doctors I see aren't from a Center of Excellence, but I love them and the nurses there. I know most people say go to a Center of Excellence, but for some people that just isn't an option. There are travel costs and some insurances won't pay for the doctor visits. There's also the question about when to start a TKI. I'm not a doctor and I'm not that knowledgeable about those drugs, but I don't understand why they say don't take it till it's compromising an organ. I feel you should stop it from growing before it gets to that point. I was talking to a lady on the MTC site and she told me her doctors had advised her to start taking them, but she refused. She said she wished she had listened because she wouldn't have had all the problems she was having today from the tumors growing.

I don't know what's right or wrong, but I just feel you should do what you and your doctors think is best. I like the saying, "You drive your own bus."

I joined the MTC Facebook page to find out more information about the Caprelsa. I've learned a lot from this page. In addition to information, there's also a lot of support from people who share their experiences. I never realized how many people suffered from this disease. I also didn't realize how different this disease is from any other. It's really hard to compare your calcitonin or CEA or metastases with anyone else. The calcitonin and CEA can differ from one lab to another. It's amazing how many people have lived years with this disease, with little to no recurrence, and then some people have had a lot of complications. If you're a newbie, just know you aren't in this journey alone. You'll have good days and bad days, and that's okay.

Remember to take of yourself.

Obsession With Uncertainty

By Kerri Remmel

Medullary thyroid cancer captured my consciousness and has not let go since I was given the diagnosis three months ago.

I read scientific journal articles before surgery that used words like "recurs," "incurable," and "lung, bone and liver metastases." I heard my MTC medical team at MD Anderson say "microscopic mets," read my abdominal CT scan results with "lesions concerning for . . ." and "plan to repeat imaging in six months." I think I'm supposed to adjust to this and move on. But I'm not good with uncertainty. Until now I've only revealed my obsession with this uncertain incurable cancer to my two soul mates.

My "new normal" of hypoparathyroidism is annoying, to say the least. Since my total thyroidectomy two months ago I have a hoarse voice, occasional swallowing difficulty, tingling paresthesias that come and go, muscle weakness and spasms, and even the famous Chvostek's sign (facial twitch), which I learned about in medical school but never thought I'd be the patient with it.

The Facebook support group of Meddies keeps me connected and unashamed of my obsession. I can check in each day with my new band of brothers and sisters, some of whom have lived with MTC for 20 years. I am connected with people who have MTC, and I have never even laid eyes on any of them. Reading their stories keeps me grounded. I am one of them. But I've got it easy compared to many, at least for now. I plan to meet many of them at the annual ThyCA conference in October.

I'm a new Meddie. Or am I? I wonder just how long I've had MTC? I had a biopsy without ultrasound guidance more than 15 years ago by an endocrinologist in her office. Results were negative, and I never thought about it again until my new PCP insisted on an ultrasound. She would not let me blow it off. I was grateful for her insistence. The ultrasound guided biopsy was performed at the University of Louisville with expertise and compassion. The nurse in radiology offered to hold my hand for support, and I took her up on it.

But I decided to find an MTC Center of Excellence, strongly recommended by my wise 90-year-old mother, so I chose MD Anderson. Every aspect of every event was played out with excellence there. And the team leader, Dr. Gary Clayman, was a phenomenon. I hung on to every syllable he uttered. I should know better, but with so much uncertainty built in to the diagnosis, I needed someone to rely on who had seen a gazillion patients with this disease. He is it.

The endocrinologist assigned to me, Dr. Habra, gave the "microscopic mets" news (based on calcitonin and CEA levels) with thoughtful compassion. He taught me more about how the disease spreads in some people and how they look at calcitonin doubling times for predicting tumor recurrence. And the MDA laboratory was unbelievable, with a huge waiting room full of people that turned over so quickly. In and out in 10 minutes. I must have been stuck 25 times while there for assessments, pre-op and post-op care, and never had a bruise on my arms. How does that happen? I'm either a bionic woman or they are that good.

I wonder what the survival rate is for T2N2MX? I guess it's too early to stage.

None of us knows how our lives will play out. Or how long we have to live. As I've told my soul mates, my life should not be measured by a length of time or a "survival rate," anyway. My life should be measured by the depth of my convictions, by my deeds, good or bad, by what difference I have made. In the end, that's what matters.

Each person with cancer must learn her own approach to transforming cancer-consciousness into cancer-subconsciousness so she may "carefully capture the minutes of her life, and live them." (Thank you, Teresa Fountain.) I'm not there yet. Cancer is still very much in the forefront. I want to make every moment count. Who doesn't?

Cancer does give me a greater appreciation of moments in everyday life. I notice moments of kindness more than ever, and cherish them. I notice negativism more, and fiercely reject it rather than patiently wait for it to submerge.

Cancer brings out truth, too. My sons opened up to me post-op and revealed their feelings of love and of their acceptance of my life. My sister and soul mate, Carol, has ways of bringing out the best in people. Crazy how that is. It took getting cancer to allow the truth to be revealed.

I am so grateful my diagnosis came after my kids were grown. They're in their twenties. I thank God that my genetics tests were negative for RET. What about my Meddie brothers and sisters who have young children? My heart aches for them.

I want MTC to stand down. I realize that it won't disappear, but it needs to fade into subconsciousness. Maybe it will move into the background after the follow-up scans at six months post-op. Or maybe not. As I write, I feel a power over MTC. I am facing it head on, but I have no idea where I'm headed. I've always set goals, strategically mapped out plans, and worked hard to achieve them. MTC is the greatest challenge yet, because I can't map out a solid plan yet.

So at three months from diagnosis and two months from TT I think about this cancer most of the time, but I'm okay. Not where I want to be, but grateful to have amazing love and support, a dynamite group of colleagues at work, a great medical team of experts at MDA, and a new family of Meddies.

Writing this initial report has helped me label this stage of my cancer journey *Obsession with Uncertainty*.

Diarrhea – The BIG D

By J. Doe

I was visiting my family in Pennsylvania one summer. One sister had decided that we'd all have a cookout at her house. Mom made potato salad, I made a veggie tray, the other sister brought chicken to grill, and my brother brought wine and beer. The hostesses made steaks, corn on the cob, and grilled carrots.

We were enjoying ourselves and the beautiful evening in a gorgeously landscaped back yard when *it* happened.

I tried running into the house, but there was brown liquid and grainy solids running down my leg. Complete embarrassment for me. Here I was, suffering a side effect of Medullary Thyroid Cancer that up until that point I had managed to keep secret. No one knew how often I discarded panties in public restrooms and went "commando." No one knew the shame of walking into a public restroom and making a huge mess and not being well enough or not having the right products to clean up the mess while waiting for the person in the next stall to leave. It was the hardest part for me. I could, after the first few months, accept that I would be dying soon. What I couldn't accept was that I never knew when or where the "Big D" would hit. Did I want to start wearing Depends at 47? No, they cause a rash, a painful, itchy rash.

But this time, at this wonderful family outing, my secret was *out*! My family was wonderful. My sisters have a gate connecting their backyards, which made part of it easy. My sister and brother-in-law moved the party over to their yard while my sister-in-law started washing the deck. My sister got a towel to hold between my legs while I walked upstairs to their bathroom. She helped me get undressed and threw my clothes into her own washer. My Mom drove to the drugstore for Imodium and then to her house for a change of clothes. I just sat on the toilet crying embarrassed tears.

Mom came back with medicine and clothing. I took a shower. Then we all joined the rest of the party. I was no longer willing to eat or drink anything for fear that the same thing would happen again. I apologized to all, explaining that it was a side effect of my particular cancer. Yes, it had happened before, and would happen again. I explained that I had yet to find a medication that would control it.

This was absolutely, positively, the worst night of my life! I had just had a major accident in front of a group of people whom I knew intimately, including my in-laws!

The good news was that my very compassionate sister-in-law, worked as a drug rep for a company that had just introduced a cholesterol medication. It was a non-statin and worked entirely in the digestive system. The one drawback it had was that it caused constipation. She gave me a few samples to take home, as well as an information packet for my doctor.

I took the stuff to my physician, who had me do a whole gastrointestinal workup to determine that my diarrhea was indeed caused entirely by my cancer. As I had a relative who worked for the company, I got my medication for free. Through a process of experimentation, I discovered that two to three of these pills every day made my life accident-free again. Even after my sister-in-law changed jobs, I continued to take these lovely pills once a day.

I haven't had an "accident" since.

The "Big D"

By Bill Prentice

During my diarrhea research, I discovered that the medical profession had already classified human feces into seven categories. This is very useful when discussing your outputs and frequencies. Personally, I went from type 1-3 every couple of days (childhood through age 40+), then from 4 through 7 in fairly rapid succession (age 45-50). During the worst of times I was suffering through weeks of type 7 with an hourly frequency, which put me at grave risk for low electrolytes and malnutrition. Food was flying through me completely undigested. I lost a total of 47 pound in six months and was hospitalized several times for severe dehydration, electrolyte imbalance, and other life-threatening side effects of uncontrolled diarrhea. Fortunately my health care team was able to keep me full of potassium and other needed chemicals, and got the diarrhea under control. Today I am happily creating type 4 feces, once or twice a day, and regaining the weight I had lost.

Google on Bristol Stool Chart.

It is quite simple and easy to understand.

People in the medullary thyroid cancer/multiple endocrine neoplasm (MEN) community understand at a glance the meaning of the term *The Big D*. This, in fact, refers to diarrhea. Now, what does thyroid cancer have to do with diarrhea?

Both medullary thyroid cancer (MTC) and multiple endocrine neoplasm (MEN) affect your digestive system. In fact, looking back over my own case, I had gastrointestinal issues long before my stage 4c medullary thyroid cancer was diagnosed. Between 1999 and 2003 I had two full bowel obstructions, resulting in two separate hospitalizations. Between those events, my digestive pattern changed dramatically.

Ever since childhood I had been a constipated person, but in my mid-40s, that condition began to change. The texture, condition, color, smell, and amount of gas behind my excrement began to change, but not in a consistent manner. One "event" could produce bile green stool, tan stool, liquid-only stool, or "rocks." Several trips to a gastroenterologist and lots of invasive testing proved nothing. I finally accepted this as some "new normal" state. It was manageable, and I was busy with a family and responsible job that required lots of interesting international travel. So with one eye out for the international toilet sign, I moved on, so to speak.

However, in 2005 I was diagnosed with sporadic medullary thyroid cancer. Upon diagnosis my calcitonin scores were 7580 (standard is <10) and CEA of 256, where it should be near zero. I had a pretty well entrenched case of medullary thyroid cancer. In researching this disease, I discovered that the calcitonin was the culprit. According to Wikipedia:

> The major clinical symptom of metastatic medullary thyroid carcinoma is diarrhea; occasionally a patient will have flushing episodes. Both occur particularly with liver metastasis, and either symptom may be the first manifestation of the disease. The flushing that occurs in medullary thyroid carcinoma is indistinguishable from that associated with carcinoid syndrome. In MTC, the flushing, diarrhea, and itching (pruritus) are all caused by elevated levels of calcitonin gene products (calcitonin or calcitonin gene-related peptide). Alternatively, the flushing and diarrhea observed in carcinoid syndrome is caused by elevated levels of circulating serotonin.

So Meddies (the name medullary thyroid cancer patients have chosen to call themselves) tend to talk a *lot* about "the Big D" and report some terribly embarrassing close calls (or worse). Sort of Meddie gallows humor. These events (or near events) became critical for me in terms of my employment. I eventually took a disability retirement discharge from what I considered to be the absolute best job I've ever had, at the absolute best company where I could ever have worked. A sad decision, but necessitated by my condition.

I will spare you those details, as I'm sure similar stories will appear elsewhere in this tome. But I will walk you through the mechanism by which MTC/MEN uses calcitonin and other peptides to mess up your day.

Calcitonin is produced directly by the medullary thyroid cancer cells as they grow in the thyroid, spread into the lymph system, and travel throughout the body. Once medullary thyroid cancer metastasizes (spreads outside the thyroid area of the neck), it often metastasizes to the liver. These liver metastases cause the liver to start producing increased levels of other peptides that also affect digestion. This is often the first sign to the patient that something is wrong. Diarrhea, flushing (hot flashes/sweats) and general fatigue are the first clues. But these are so mundane and sporadic they are often ignored or put on the back burner. That is, until the diarrhea becomes unbearable. Once the doctors figured out that my gastric issues were calcitonin related, we were off to the races!

There are several mechanisms used to fight the *Big D* monster. Some are traditional diarrhea controls such as over-the-counter drugs like Imodium and prescriptions like Lomotil. These drugs basically slow down the intestinal tract (because the calcitonin and other peptides have it running full steam ahead!) If these don't work, other approaches try to attach and flush through the calcitonin, allowing it to do its deed. This approach uses drugs originally designed to capture and flush through cholesterol, so if you have high cholesterol *and* medullary thyroid cancer-related diarrhea, this could really work for you. These drugs are bile acid sequestrants like:

- Cholestyramine (Questran®)
- Colesevelam (Welchol™)
- Colestipol (Colestid®)

If none of these approaches work, the heavy hitter is deodorized tincture of opium (DTO). This is just what it sounds like. It is opium dissolved in alcohol (a tincture). The term *deodorized* refers to the chemical removal of some of the more narcotic (addictive) qualities of whole opium extract. This is a very effective drug, but must be used with extreme caution. It is typically dosed in drops, as a teaspoonful is enough to be fatal. It is also still somewhat addictive and can be subject to intentional or even unintentional abuse. It works by significantly slowing your digestive system's motility (the movements your intestines and colon make to move food through your system). Patients must be careful to not *stop* their digestion by overusing DTO. This will land you back in the ER with a bowel obstruction. Full circle from where I started!

The Chosen One

By Joyce Johnson

Since my diagnosis of MTC, I've been afforded the "luxury" of having more time to write letters to friends and family. The ability to reconnect with some people, while maintaining and/or growing relationships with others has truly been cathartic and in some cases therapeutic for me. It's definitely cheaper and more convenient than weekly therapy visits.

Just recently, one of my dear friends asked a big question that allowed me to dig a little deeper and come to terms with what having cancer means to me. Of course, lots of thoughts popped into my head. But what she wanted me to zero in on was to talk about the difference between being the one with the cancer versus watching a loved one having to deal with it firsthand. So, she asked me specifically how I feel about this and went on to say that when she was dealing with her own diagnosis of uterine cancer she actually felt a sense of empowerment because she knew she would not rest until she beat this or died trying. Period. In a way, being the one with The Cancer gave her a new sense of being and a renewed sense of direction. Don't get me wrong, it's not like she needed this jolt in her life, but she's a very strong woman and loves her son beyond measure and she knew without a doubt that it would be a lot easier for her to deal with cancer in her life, as long as it was in her body and not in her son or her sister or anyone else that held a piece of her heart. Yes, she and I are very good and close friends but as much as we love each other we are separate enough to know that we are not in each other's tight circle and our friendship is strong enough to handle the truth. Which is cancer and it is bound to happen to a certain number of people and the odds were that someone in her family and someone in my family would be chosen. And we both agree that while we are not ecstatic about having a diagnosis of cancer, we are more than ok with our immediate family members not being afflicted with it.

I say afflicted and not affected because the fact of the matter is, everyone is affected to some degree. That's one of the sureties of cancer, it affects all. You don't have to actually get it to have some kind of reaction to it, adverse or otherwise.

Now back to her question. Am I glad that this cancer is in my body and not in my husband's or son's body? It took me a nanosecond to respond. I say unequivocally, bar none, hands down, with no reservations and without hesitation, yes. If cancer had to come into our lives and it was destined to pick one of the three of us, I am happy to be the "The Chosen One". And no it's not a martyrdom thing. It's more about still feeling like I have a bit of control in my life. In other words, God forbid if our 26 year old son turned up with cancer, it would be a million times worse for me than just having cancer myself. And even as I write this, my heart breaks for those in our ThyCa Family who know exactly what these words mean. They not only have MTC, they have children and nieces and nephews and other close family members who also have MTC. And they know deep down in their bones how much this hurts. Please understand what I am trying to say. None of this is easy. None of this is good. None of this is right. But it is a truth in our lives. Cancer is a reality that we all have to deal with and I can only speak from what I know. I'm in no way trying to compare or contrast anyone else's personal experience. I'm doing my best to answer my dear friend's personal, heartfelt question to me.

In my letter responding to my friend, I shared the above thoughts with her and I went on to say that I'm the type that if I must ride on this 'hell-bound' train, I prefer to be in the driver's seat and not be a passenger. I guess that's where the control issues come in. I feel if I make a mistake, it will be on me. I take full responsibility for my actions. If I choose a certain type of treatment, or choose to see different doctors, or if I choose to take the wait and watch approach, the common theme here is I got to choose. And getting to choose is important to me. If my choices don't pan out as I planned, I will pay the price for my decisions. And that's not to say that my decisions won't affect my family and friends, no not at all. But, I truly believe they know my heart and they know I'm not scared and they know I handle these kinds of life challenges better when I'm hit between the eyes rather than a glancing blow. That's just the way I am. I don't do anything half-assed and (un)fortunately neither does Cancer.

Who knows? Maybe Cancer and I are cut from the same cloth and we will learn something from each other. I know this adversary has already taught me a lot and I don't plan on going down without teaching it a thing or two. There's an old saying that goes, "Keep your friends close but your enemies closer". In conclusion, I'd like to say that being the "The Chosen One" is the best option for me and I invite my cancer to snuggle up close and prepare to bring it on!

Relearning How To Hope

By HJC

It was the day after my 25th birthday when I drove myself to the hospital to have a neck ultrasound. It was the first in what turned out to be a series of tests that eventually led to a diagnosis of medullary thyroid carcinoma, a disease I had never even heard of until that fall. My disease was Stage IV, sporadic, extremely invasive in the neck, with metastases to the mediastinum, lungs, and liver. For a while I had thought it was papillary carcinoma, the "first kind" of thyroid cancer, the 90 percent kind, the easier-to-treat kind. I had prepared myself for the possibility of cancer, and when it was confirmed, expected that surgery and radioactive iodine would provide a cure. A follow-up blood test revealed that my calcitonin, the telltale MTC tumor marker, was staggeringly high. There was no doubt. This was not papillary.

That night, as I drove to a friend's house to share the news, I remember weeping, crying out to God, lost, unsure what to do or how I was going to bear this burden. All I could hold on to through the tears was a desperate prayer, "I will trust you, and I will trust you, and I will wait on you."

It takes a long time for traumatic news to sink in. I remember lying in the hospital bed after surgery. Everything was new. My experience at hospitals up to that point had been minimal. Despite years of misdiagnosed symptoms, I had not felt sick when my surgeon solemnly and gently told me the news four days earlier. Now, lying there propped up against a mountain of pillows, Johnny unflatteringly covering my small frame, hair matted, dizzy from the pain meds, with a bandage covering the gaping scar on my neck—*now* I felt sick. Weak, sore, unable to talk above a whisper, barely able to eat or drink, and all of a sudden I realized: This is the rest of my life. It's not a bump in the road. It *is* the road. That was the moment when reality started setting in.

I had been told not to think about this battle in terms of a cure. What they were hoping for was "long-term stability." Over the next several months, as I began an oral chemotherapy regimen and had more scans, I tried to remind myself that stable was good. But stable didn't feel good. Stable felt second-rate. Stable felt unfair, unjust even. It wasn't good enough, especially when it came at the cost of debilitating fatigue. For a long time tears of exhaustion became my daily companion. Was it even worth it? Give me a goal and I'd work hard, endure any difficulty along the way to reach it. What was my goal in fighting this cancer? There was no goal. I was in limbo.

It's nearly impossible to describe my dissatisfaction at my situation, this idea of no cure, except to say that it felt a little like Mike and Sully in *Monsters, Inc.* being banished to the Himalayas, frantically opening the door to get back to the factory, only to find swirling snow on the other side. There was no going back.

I think that's part of the injustice I felt—the feeling of no control, the fact that something colossal had happened to me and I had absolutely no part in the decision, no chance to prepare, and no hope of reversal. I wanted to bang on the factory door until someone opened it and let me back in. Acceptance felt like resignation. It felt like giving up, and I couldn't pull the two concepts apart in my mind. Now at last the distinction between acceptance and resignation is clearer. How it became clear, I don't know. It takes time. Time and the grace of God in a million forms.

Slowly I grew accustomed to new routines, and to the things that were scary becoming familiar and blending into the daily, weekly, monthly rhythms of life. Now, I no longer feel anxious as I lie motionless, listening to the banging, tapping, and beeping of the MRI machine. I'm used to the prodding and poking of needles and the spreading burning sensation of the I.V. contrast. I can rattle off my medical record number as if it were my phone number. I've gotten used to the strange thoughts that come into my mind. For instance, when my pastor asked in a sermon, "Where do you see yourself in thirty years?" my first thought was, "I don't know if I'll be alive in thirty years." I didn't used to think those kinds of thoughts, but when cancer enters your mental landscape, it changes everything.

It's only been a year and a half, and I can't remember anymore what it's like not to have cancer, or visit the doctor only once or twice a year, or live an entire day without once thinking about death. My mental landscape has changed drastically, and there's nothing I can do about it. But I know I have come a long way when occasionally I laugh over a thought that would probably have made me cry a year ago. The other day I offered my roommate a bite of my food. Colds were going around, so before she took the fork she asked, "Are you sick?" My response: "Define sick." We couldn't stop laughing. Strange thoughts. Familiar thoughts.

Coming to a place of more healing and rest, I find that I don't think these thoughts any less often than I used to, but now they hold less power over me. I'm relearning how to hope. Sometimes I can't see to take the next step and sometimes I'm robbed of the will to keep moving forward entirely. And then after an eternity of stumbling, I look back and trace the footprints of grace.

I'm young, but I feel old in my suffering. I know it's not over. I'm trying to learn to sit with the questions and live in the tension between joy and sorrow and—in the end, I hope and trust—joy.

*I can't remember a trial or a pain
He did not recycle to bring me gain
I can't remember one single regret
In serving God only, and trusting His hand
All I have need of, His hand will provide
He's always been faithful to me.*

Sara Groves

A Caregiver's Journal: In Rare Meddie Form

By Debbie Bambenek

How do you put into words how this rare, incurable cancer has changed our lives? From a wife, mom, and caregiver's perspective, I can only tell you from my heart.

From the beginning of this journey, November 2011, there has been fear, denial, hope, courage, strength, joy, pain, undeniable love, and pride. This is to name a short list of emotions.

We have been affected, yes. Have we felt the walls crumbling in around us? Most certainly.

But I am here to tell you, this will *not* pull us in. Nope, it will only make us stronger! Our God has a reason for everything. We may never know the reasons as to why, but we have learned to live with strength, hope, faith, and courage. One step, one day at a time.

I started a journal in the early days of this journey, and I'll share pieces of those days with you.

12-16-11

So much to absorb in so little time. We had a rough day of tears, fears, and deep conversation on this, the third trip of the week to Gunderson. Rich is so unselfish, caring, loving, do anything–for–anybody kind of man. My dream come true, the love of my life. Why us? Why him? This journey will be a challenge for us all. The support has been amazing already. It's so overwhelming! My days are running into nights and I'm in a haze.

The cell rings and then the landline. I just can't keep up! We're working on taking it day-by-day, not looking too deeply or coming to our own conclusions. I am so grateful for the genuine care from family and friends.

Monday will be busy and tiring, I'm sure! One week until Christmas, my favorite holiday, which will mean so much more this year.

12-17-11

The day started a bit calm. I am doing my best to keep his spirits up. He's so strong, but always the worrier. There's no turning back, all we can do is fight forward.

I set up a Caring Bridge site while Rich napped. He had a pretty restless night, which means I did, too. This will calm down as soon as we have a plan. We'll kill this cancer with positivity! Get your rest, Dear Rich, we're going into this like gangbusters! Full speed ahead! Work your wonders, Dear God.

12-18-11

Almost a full week since all of this started. We pray we can complete this soon. We went to see Rich's parents, having not seen or talked to them since the diagnosis. The visit was necessary, I felt. The family was able to gather to give Rich love and encouragement before we go into this next week. I'm pretty positive, but scared for him. I am behind him, 100 percent of the way. Tomorrow is a new day and a new challenge, and we're ready to take it on.

12-19-11

Biopsy on lymph nodes, vocal cord and chest x-ray were all done today. His surgeon gave him the calcitonin levels, which are 10,500. The level we hoped to be under was 400. So that means we need to head to their other facility for a CT scan to see if there has been spreading. Chest x-ray was clear and all other tests have been good so far. He's going into this as healthy as he can be. That is a blessing. He looks so sad. I talked to him and told him no matter what, he needed to be open with me so I can help him. I don't know what he's dealing with, but I am his other half. When he hurts, I hurt. I love him so much that taking care of him is easy. He may have the cancer and I can never imagine going through that, but I have to be his strength when he can't. I have the kids to protect, let alone myself.

Please be with us, Dear Lord.

12-20-11

We have yet another hurdle. The CT scan showed a spot on his liver. That would be the third biopsy. This surgeon left us with the option to test or to leave it and watch it. It's a no-brainer. Test it for peace of mind. Everything else is good and ready to go. Feeling that if the doctors are not okay with that spot, they would have forced us into a biopsy. So we are viewing it as a precautionary step.

So much info to absorb.

Seven days before surgery with 2-5 weeks of recovery. Then I think they will do radiation. So that will be after complete healing. And *that* will be a reassurance that they got it *all*. (Later: As we know, that is *not* an option for MTC patients, and he did not have this done.)

All infected areas or anything suspicious will be taken as well. Leaning a lot on God these days.

12-21-11

Wow! What a long day, starting at 4:30am and off to Gunderson to prep and wait for a 9:30am biopsy. Our registration was over two hours long because they didn't have a doctor's order for the genetic blood test. Which means, for us, another visit to the geneticist to see if he carries MEN, which causes the cancer. Hopefully that's done before surgery on Tuesday.

Time for this to be over, it's exhausting.

12-22-11

Sad day in our house. We are now dealt another challenge in our battle. The spot on his liver is cancer. Thank you, Devil, thank you so much, but our fight and battle is on and I'm sorry to say, we have a bigger army, and we are going to kick some major butt.

We are starting over tomorrow and you can burn in love, prayer and hope. Dear God, please give us strength to get through this.

12-23-11

It was so good to gather with family and take this off our minds for a bit. We continue to pray for strength and feel the abundance of love from friends and family. So grateful for everyone and having God on our side. It's a half hour from Christmas Eve. God be a blessing to us all.

12-24-11

What a nice, wonderful and refreshing evening! It was great being with family and laughing, after tears! God, please be always with him, every step of the way. At church tonight, not only was it all decorated so magically, it was very touching and straight to the point of Christmas. After mass, my Brother-in-Law asked the pastor to pray over Rich. We gathered around him and we all cried feeling the power of God working His way through us. It was a wonder. Thank you, God, for showing us the way. All troubles seemed to melt away this magical evening. It was good for all of us.

Happy Birthday, Jesus!

12-31-11

So much has happened since Christmas. The surgery went well, but another *slam* as an MRI was taken and he has more spots all over his liver. Next stop, Mayo.

Dear God, get us out of this, please.

One step at a time, that's all we can do. He's on our side and we'll get through this with a new perspective on life. Just wishing what's coming won't make it so. Positivity is our goal. With the help, love and forgiveness of all of our sins, from God.

(In the meantime, Rich had been seen at Mayo with Dr. Bible. He started him on Caprelsa to slow the tumor growth and possibly shrink the smaller ones.)

The kids were tested for the RET gene as Rich was diagnosed as the index case of MEN2A. Our daughter (who at the time was 20) was negative. Our son (15 years old at the time) was positive. We got him started right away at Mayo. Going into this with knowledge that it's just the gene doesn't mean he has cancer. All blood tests were normal and ultrasound was clear. Set up for surgery, and it went very well. But when we spoke to the surgeon, Dr. Thompson, he noted that micro Medullary was found, contained to the thyroid. No other spots were seen.

What? My son now has cancer, one week from his 16th birthday? What did this mean?

We can deal with it. God has prepared us well. Rich's diagnosis has saved our son from going through what we did. Our son has fared very well. CEA and calcitonin are undetectable to normal. We are on a watch and wait with a pheo that is too tiny to remove as of yet. He will be on a yearly basis for labs and 24-hour urine test every two years, face to face with his endocrinologist, Dr. Young. Blessed there, so to say.

7-22-12

Eight months into this and still fighting the battle. My love for this man grows stronger each day. I felt driven to write in the journal, Caring Bridge isn't the place for my personal feelings. The weekend was a tough one to get through. Many ups and downs. Rich is tiring of the "D," which has been a daily issue for the three and one-half years we've been on this journey. We worry about weight and nutrition. We'll do whatever is needed for survival. I shed a lot of tears this weekend and tried to shout out to God for peace and calmness right away. I know he'll provide our needs. I have so many regrets for the days, months, etc., that I have taken our love for granted. He is the love of my life, my dream come true. And I cannot stand that he is going through this. I love him so much.

Dear God, watch over us. Please take away the cancer, please allow for Rich and me to live healthy and strong, to watch our beautiful children become successful and happy. To witness to the loves of their lives that You have been preparing for them. And, too, from that love we'll see our grandbabies, their flesh and blood. I want to be strong and healthy alongside of Rich, to be able to play and laugh and take care of these beautiful creations. Please keep us growing in faith and help us to live in eternal life with you, Dear Lord.

2015

Much has happened since that last entry. I have become active in our new family, the MTC support site. They all have helped me to learn that we are not alone in this journey. I have personally met another meddie and his wife. And I have become friends with so many others. I have witnessed death and cried so many tears for these families. I pray, cry, cheer and love, with each and every one of them. God has taken too many home, too early. With those deaths, we each have another angel to guide us through our days. I have learned to cope with and to accept the many challenges we have faced and possibly can face in the road ahead.

Rich is now on his second chemo (Cometriq) and it's working except for some gallbladder issues. The first one (Calpresa) was working for two years, except for a few months off this past summer (2014). This one has also started strong. It was a long healing process because of the radiation to a couple areas.

With each passing day there is a "new normal."

The past six months have been like a retreat. He has heard "stable" on the last two doctor visits, three months apart. This word is exactly what we needed to hear. It's been quite the ride, and we're doing it as gracefully as we can. Making every minute count. Never taking life for granted, even seconds.

Much too short.

Live. Laugh. Love. God bless us all!

A Mom's Journey With MTC

By Sharon Ferraro

My daughter was diagnosed with sporadic Medullary Thyroid Cancer (MTC) on April 6, 2010, at the age of 17. She was a junior in high school. It has been a unique journey for me, and I never imagined how inspiring, spiritual and stressful it could be.

And still is.

My personal journey started months before Nicole's diagnosis. She was complaining of a stiff and sore neck in late summer of 2009, which continued through the end of the year and into early 2010. Our chiropractor was trying to help her, and at times she seemed to improve. During the fall of 2009, I read an article about how we should live our lives like a GPS, not judging things but just "recalculating." I thought it was a great way to look at life.

Then over the New Year's holiday I was praying for my annual Guidepost word/phrase to be with me through the year and the word "recalculating" came to me. I had actually forgotten about the article. I really felt that God put that word in my heart, so I decided to keep that word for 2010. Little did I know that Nicole would be diagnosed with cancer within four months!

When the diagnosis was made, and throughout my journey, the theme of "recalculating" has definitely helped me. We should not judge what happens to us because nothing is really good or bad, right or wrong. It's just what it is. We recalculate, adjust our path, and keep going.

When Nicole was diagnosed on April 6, 2010 it was two days after Easter. On Easter, Nicole was sent a Bible verse from her Young Life Leader that also made a great impact on our perspective of her cancer diagnosis. John 3:16 was sent to her ("For God so loved the world, that He gave His only begotten Son, that whoever believes in Him shall not perish, but have eternal life."), and she asked me to write it down so she could look it up later. Her dad then told her what the verse was about, so she handed me back the small piece of paper on which she had written "John 3:16." Somehow I kept that paper and put it on my desk at home. I don't remember making a decision to do that. I will come back to that paper soon.

Nicole's journey with testing, appointments and discussions regarding her diagnosis took about six weeks, which was after our chiropractor had told us in mid-February 2010 that he could not help her. Nicole had begun complaining of a sore spot in her collarbone area, along with a stiff neck. Our chiropractor said "This could be lymph node related or thyroid." I thought he was not accurate in bringing up the thyroid, given how far away it was from the sore spot, but we did go to our general doctor, who ordered an ultrasound of the sore spot. She couldn't feel any lumps in Nicole's neck, and the ultrasound showed a normal-looking lymph node (Note: at this time she did not ask for an ultrasound of the neck, which should have been done). We then were sent to an orthopedic doctor for an x-ray, which was normal, and he thought she needed a test for mononucleosis, which was negative.

We were then sent to a surgeon's office who said, "Well, cancer doesn't usually hurt." He ordered an MRI of the neck, which came back "cloudy" on the right side of the thyroid. We then were told to go to a doctor for a fine needle biopsy of the sore lymph node in the collarbone area.

Nicole prepped with Valium, and the doctor then decided he didn't need to do the biopsy after all because it felt normal and not a problem. He told us to come back when we had something else for him to biopsy. I called back our general doctor, who suggested the ultrasound on Nicole's neck.

All these tests and doctor visits took about six weeks. The ultrasound was done and the diagnostic staff person came out afterwards to talk with us. He said he didn't usually talk directly with patients, but he saw what we had been through. He wanted us to know that Nicole had a 2cm nodule on the right side of her thyroid and needed to talk with a surgeon, as this could possibly be cancer. The surgeon then had us go back for a fine needle biopsy, which took place on April 10, 2010, two days after Easter and our John 3:16 message.

The doctor conducted the biopsy, went to the next room to review under the microscope, and came back with, "You have thyroid cancer. And actually, you have a rare kind that could be hereditary, and you're going to need surgery."

After we came home and cried/talked for a little while, Nicole actually wanted to go to her high school to watch a soccer game! She wanted to keep going, which astonished me. I had told her that God would help us through this and that she shouldn't let this stop her, but I didn't think she would understand so quickly! I went to my desk where my chair was facing opposite the desk. I sat and turned around, and thought, "What do I do now?" As I faced my desk, that piece of paper with John 3:16 on it was the first thing I saw. I got such a chill, and I felt like if I really believed that we were going to heaven, then everything would be okay. I felt she belonged to God, and I was her caregiver. I now had to "walk the talk." It was a very powerful experience.

Nicole's surgery was done at Johns Hopkins University Hospital a month later. She had the RET test, which was negative. Her calcitonin was around 10,500 and CEA was 262. We were blessed with two very experienced thyroid cancer surgeons and an MTC specialist/endocrinologist. Even with their skills and scans, they were not prepared for what the surgery showed. Nicole had cancer that had spread beyond the thyroid and beyond the lymph nodes (28 of 36 nodes were cancerous on the right side, and all stuck together). It appeared on a nerve leading to the side of her face, a nerve to her right vocal cord and a nerve to the right side of her diaphragm, as well as cancer in the shoulder muscle. Scans showed spots in her mediastinum and lungs too, but those could not be addressed during this first surgery, which took about eight hours.

At about the five-hour mark during surgery I was told that one of the surgeons wanted to talk to me. I thought they had completed surgery early. Boy, was I wrong! She came to say that the cancer had spread well beyond what she had ever seen. She asked me if they could remove the nerve to the right vocal cord because there was cancer on it. She knew that Nicole loved to sing every day, so she wanted to check with me. However, for me it sounded like a question that didn't need to be asked. The cancer had to be removed. I asked the surgeon if she was asking because Nicole was going to die anyway and that's why it was up to me. She really didn't have an answer, so I told her to remove the nerve. That moment was the deepest despair I had ever felt.

After surgery, many meetings took place regarding future treatment options, since there were no chemotherapies available at that time. After much confusion and stress it was decided that she would have radiation on the right side of her neck due to there not being clear margins after surgery on her trachea and in her shoulder muscle area. It was certainly a challenge for us to learn all we could on our own so we could understand the doctors and the options. Our Hopkins doctor (Dr. Doug Ball) had some data about radiation on microscopic cells, but we realized that much of what was possible wasn't clear-cut or recommended. They were just ideas.

We didn't go with the first option with a highly respected radiation oncologist who said radiation had to be done on her entire neck and that she should have her wisdom teeth out beforehand. Nicole didn't want that, and we didn't want it, either. We decided on radiation on the right side only.

Dr. Ball prepared us for the news that the cancer could grow more, and perhaps to other areas due to what was found in surgery. We found a natural supplement called TBL-12 that Nicole started taking before her radiation treatments began in October 2010 because it was highly recommended by another mom whose son had MTC, and she knew the only distributor of it who lived near her. We decided to try it for three months, since we felt things were so out of our control at the time. After that time frame scans were stable, so she continued for six more months. As Nicole continued to remain stable, we kept taking it. She continued taking the supplement and was very stable for four years. She also had three annual vocal cord injections and in 2013 she had an implant, but no more cancer growth. In 2014 she didn't take TBL-12 daily for three trips in the first half of that year. In July 2014 another spot was found in her lower left lung, which was partially collapsing that area and needed immediate treatment.

Again, specialists didn't know what the best treatment was. We had to make our decision as we were learning all we could. First, one of two new oral chemotherapies was recommended. Then a biopsy was done to try and confirm the cancer, but it didn't work. Chemotherapy was discussed again. I reached out to Dr. Tuttle at Sloan Kettering, since he had monitored Nicole's case (in partnership with Dr. Ball). After discussions and appointments it was decided to have lung surgery at Sloan to remove the lower left lobe. Surgery took place in late September, but unfortunately the surgery didn't work. The cancer spot had spread over into the upper lobe and the surgeon didn't want to remove the entire left lung. The discussion immediately went back to the oral chemotherapy options. It was heartbreaking and stressful to keep changing the options, but in my mind I tried to keep "recalculating." It helped to not judge or label what was happening; just do it.

It was decided Nicole would begin taking Caprelsa, which was started on October 11. Her counts reduced a lot by January, and her scans also showed reductions. Her calcitonin was 750 and her CEA was 115, which was a big change from a previous calcitonin of 23,897 and CEA of 143 on September 30. We were so happy with these numbers (although many reading these numbers might not be). We are now awaiting the next batch of scans and labs on May 26.

Throughout this journey, I could not imagine all that Nicole has accomplished. She successfully graduated high school. She graduated college in four years on May 9, 2015. She started a foundation called Bite Me Cancer in September 2010 (www.bitemecancer.org) to raise research funds for Thyroid Cancer, and also to support/inspire teenagers battling cancer. The foundation continues to grow, and she continues to inspire many people.

Early in our journey, I heard a beautiful song by Laura Story called "Blessings" that still helps me. Also there is a powerful song by Kutless called "What Faith Can Do" that still helps us. We have received John 3:16 through other times in this journey, just when we have needed it. For me, this is a journey of faith as well as a journey of cancer. Every day of life is a blessing. Every experience of life is a blessing. I pray every day to have peace in this journey and to give Nicole the best possible life that God has to offer her.

Damn You, Cancer!

By Mary Belisle

Damn you, cancer!

To hell with you!

I never thought that playing with my son would lead me to hearing the words: You have cancer!

I was chasing my 14-year-old around the house, goofing off, and he jumped on the couch. I jumped, too, and his head came back and hit my throat. I felt pain right away, but thought nothing of it. After four to five days though, I called the doctor, who checked it out and said it was probably nothing, but wanted to get an ultrasound, anyway. Three days later I met my new endocrinologist, Dr. Robert Cooper. Then came another ultrasound and a needle biopsy. We talked for a bit. I told him I was the type of person who liked to be straightforward, no sugar coating anything. I asked him if he thought it was cancer, and of course he told me he wouldn't know until the biopsy came back. So I asked again, with different wording. Does it look like cancer to you from what you've seen already? He said yes. I thanked him for his honesty and made my next appointment for the results.

I read everything I could find on thyroid cancer. From what I learned, I did not want medullary or anaplastic. Those two seemed to be the ones with the worse outcome. *Please, please,* not the last two is all I kept saying as I waited. However, the results confirmed that it was thyroid cancer. *Not the last two, not the last two,* I said a few times to myself, and then asked, "So which type is it?" The doctor said medullary. "Well, okay, what should I do?" I asked. That's all I could say. He told me the first thing I needed to do was get to a place that had doctors who knew what they were doing and who treated this type of cancer often. He told me to go to MD Anderson. I fought the insurance and did just that.

I had been having trouble before diagnosis with swallowing, bad diarrhea, flushing, always being cold, freezing in the winter so bad it hurt to walk, bad night sweats. However, my blood work for thyroid function came back normal. So why did I feel like shit all the time? Nobody could figure it out, so I let it go and stopped complaining about it.

Little did I know what was brewing inside me. When I heard those words I was floored. I have three children and a husband I want to be around for! I had crying fits and figured out who was getting what if I should die from this. It was a horrible feeling.

I finally got to MD Anderson, where the tests started and ended three days later. I never had so many tests in my life. I had to get another fine needle biopsy so this hospital could also verify I had this crappy cancer. Well, in 27 minutes it was confirmed that I had it. What the hell!

You can go to hell, cancer! I hate you for doing this to my family and me!

I met with the doctors to go over my results. I would need to have a total thyroidectomy with central, bi-lateral and left neck dissection. There was a mass on my adrenal gland, a small nodule by my aorta, and a few nodules in my lungs, which told me the cancer had metastasized.

Son of a bitch! The immediate concern was having my neck surgery. I made plans for surgery and saw a genetic counselor for a blood test that would tell me if I was sporadic or hereditary.

Eighteen days later I went back for my results. *Please, please let me be sporadic, please.* "Nope," the genetic counselor said. "You have a RET mutation of C620F, which makes you MEN2A, and that means it's hereditary."

Damn it! Oh God, please don't tell me my children could have this.

Not them, please! The thought of my children having to go through this made me sick to my stomach. I went back to my hotel room, called my family to tell them the results and to tell them that they needed to be tested for this damn RET mutation.

The following day I had my surgery. Five and a half hours later, my family was told everything went well. I lost two of my parathyroids so my calcium was crashing a lot in the hospital, and as a result I had to take liquid calcium, which is the worst, ever! I had a drain in my neck that was gross as hell. It filled with blood and clear fluids and had to be emptied every couple hours. After three days I was able to go back to my hotel room. After nine days I was told I could leave Texas and return to Massachusetts, toting my drain and a half-gallon of liquid calcium. I was so happy to be going home to be with my husband and children.

I was home the next day by 3:00 pm and ready for a nap. The looks I got from strangers were hurtful. They looked at me like I was a freak. My youngest son even told a lady to stop looking at me, and said, "Maybe you should ask *why* she has a drain in her neck and steri-strips half-way across her neck." Needless to say, she turned around and stopped staring.

My next step was getting my three children tested. My youngest two, aged 14 and 23, tested positive for the mutation. My oldest son refused to get tested for more than a year. I think he was afraid to know. He finally got tested and he was *negative*! Thank God.

My 14-year-old had surgery three months after being diagnosed. His CEA and calcitonin were very low, which was great to hear. His surgery went well, but it took him more than a year to get his calcium under control. When he'd tell me his fingers and face were tingly, he would have blood work done, and sure enough, his calcium was off. It bothers him every so often, even after three and a half years. His cancer markers are undetectable as of now, and I couldn't be any happier.

My daughter had her surgery a year after she was diagnosed. She was having the flushing, the sweating, and the frequent diarrhea, but still didn't want this surgery. Her CEA and calcitonin were slightly elevated, which is never good. She was afraid of this whole surgery thing and having to live with no thyroid and having to take a replacement medication for the rest of her life. She is doing better now. Not all better, but better. Her cancer markers have gone down a little since surgery, but not below five, so it might be growing in her somewhere, and that scares me. Only time will tell what happens next.

This cancer sucks! I've heard so, so many people say that with all the cancers out there, thyroid cancer is the one to have! Bullshit! I have medullary thyroid cancer, and this is how I live on a daily basis. I take a medication every day to replace my thyroid hormone, and the dose can change at any time because my body changes, so today I might feel good. But most days I am so damn tired I can't think straight. I have diarrhea all the time, I have night sweats, and I'm cold all the time, so cold it hurts to walk because my feet are frozen. My thoughts are never clear and my body hurts around the clock. The cancer in my thyroid has been removed, but this little cancer bastard left a lot of itself in other parts of my body. It's growing in my neck again. It's growing in my liver, my spine, in my chest, by my aorta, in my lungs, and who knows where else right now. So please, please tell me what part of this damn cancer is the good part. There is NO cancer that is good. NONE!

Everyone says, well, have you had chemotherapy or radiation? And when I tell them that traditional treatments don't work for this type of cancer, they look at me like I'm lying. There are other treatments, such as pills that can help, but only after the mass is big and bothersome. It doesn't work on the cancer if it's too small. Again, the look on their faces says it all. I usually just stop there because I can see they've lost interest in the story.

I plan on putting up a fight for my children and me for as long as I have to. I refuse to be pushed around by this bastard. I pray to my God every day to thank him for letting me be here another day, to be here for my family. I'm not well, but I'm healthy spiritually, emotionally, and am loved by my family and friends so very much. I want to say thank you to them for understanding. I love them so very much.

A Day In The Life Of...

By Holly Bechard

I'm hurting tonight. My lower back and my lower abdomen both throb with that low level, constant kind of uncomfortable pain that there's no getting out from once it starts. Today my husband and I dropped our two young children off at school and once again spent the day sacrificing our time and money and mental space on the altar of living with incurable cancer.

We've been doing this a lot recently.

We had fun today. We laughed and held hands in the car. We made jokes that the genetic counselor laughed at, and found time in between appointments to eat at our favorite pancake place.

The bacon was exceptionally good today.

But we also exchanged a lot of well-known glances, ones that say, "She doesn't know about this cancer, does she?" and, "Does that mean what I think it means?" I doubt anyone notices those glances we've gotten so good at exchanging. We prayed together and we prayed alone. For peace, for healing, for courage, and for patience. We both fought back tears at certain points of the day, and on the drive home to pick up the kids, we both fought the overwhelming exhaustion that seems to usually follow a day of endless medical consultations, procedures, imaging, questioning and seeking answers to questions that have no answers. We pulled into the driveway of our precious friends who love and support our children, and us, and we sat there in the rain, summoning the strength to re-enter the normal parts of life. The backpacks and the homework and the trip to the store to buy eggs so we'd have an egg carton for tomorrow's school egg hunt and 12 small toys to fill 12 plastic eggs with. Dinner and baths and reading Llama llama and Dr Seuss. All the things I love, the things I live for. And yet, some days, like today, doing these things takes summoning energy from so deep down I think I may never find it.

Sweet husband suggests we pick up pizza for dinner and sets the table with paper plates, God bless him. We all hold hands and pray for the healing of our many friends who are also suffering from cancer. We read books and tuck those beautiful little heads into bed.

And then we check email and catch up on what we missed at work today because life is still going at full speed. I'm a nurse practitioner, and also teach, so I have messages from patients and students alike who need my attention. A patient needs refills, another's depression isn't improving even after months of aggressive treatment. Several of my students have just failed my course and are realizing how drastically this might affect their immediate future. They came looking for me but I wasn't there today. Could we schedule a meeting tomorrow? Of course, that's my job. And I love it. I really do.

But this cancer, it's taking up a lot of my time. It's taking me away from my children and my friends, from my husband at times and from my patients and students. It's exhausting and frustrating, because this cancer has been growing inside of me for at least nine years that I know about, probably longer. And while it's slow growing and I don't often have to give up more than a few days of regular life at a time to deal with its effects, it's still managing to bleed into every corner of my existence.

And days like today, I just don't know if I have the strength to keep living this double life. The "I'm great, doing great, feeling great, not afraid of dying from cancer" life. And the, "I've got cancer growing in my spine and pelvis and liver and it's starting to hurt and there's no cure and we have so many unanswered questions and so many medical bills, and we're so tired of it all" life.

But we make it. We do all the things and we give those precious blonde-headed babies one last kiss and crawl into bed, check Facebook and the weather, laugh about something funny we saw today and then turn out the lights.

Because God is good, all the time. And He calls us to love others the way he loves us. Which is impossible, but for today, we tried. We tried to show love to those who cared for us in the clinics and the hospitals, in the examining rooms and at the pancake place. We loved our kids and made sure to tell them today how proud we are of them and how much we love them.

And that's really all we can do. All that matters, anyways. Cancer is cruel, relentless and unpredictable, but I am not. And I refuse to let this disease make me something I am not. So, at least for today, I think I'm winning the battle.

When I Heard The Word Cancer

By Rae Charles

When I heard the word cancer, the biggest change in my life was that it became unpredictable. Like playing a game of Whack-a-Mole.

Between dealing with surgeries, radiation, other health issues, job loss, money issues, and learning new skills, something always needed to be dealt with. In the last four years I've learned not to count on a new normal quite yet.

January 2011. The year started off wonderfully. Our son had found the love of his life and they announced their engagement in February, our daughter was in the middle of her junior year at Georgetown, and my husband and I were anxiously looking forward to good times ahead. Both of us were in our mid-fifties, anticipating being empty nesters and spending time with each other.

The end of March changed everything. While shaving, Bruce found a knot on the side of his neck. He thought that was a little strange. Although he felt fine, he went to have it checked out by his primary doctor on March 31. His doctor concluded it was a lymph node. "You probably have an infection," he said, and prescribed ten days of antibiotics.

Coincidentally, he had a dentist appointment immediately after that appointment. The dentist told him, "I don't think that's all it is." He advised Bruce to go back to the primary and ask for a CT scan.

April 2011. The doctor scheduled the scan for April 1. We got a call later that night telling us they'd found something that needed to be looked into. We were in an oncologist's office on April 3 and she scheduled a biopsy for April 6. She said she thought the scans showed some kind of lymphoma, and depending on the results, "We'll just pop that puppy out and put you through a course of chemotherapy, and you'll probably be fine."

We left that office feeling shaky. The results came back medullary thyroid cancer (MTC), and I thank my lucky stars that the doctor's residency had been at Sloan Kettering, where she'd had the opportunity to work with this disease.

My first thought was, how long does he have? How much suffering will he go through? Can I be strong enough to help him through this? Will we get through this? I'm not ready to lose him. He won't be around for Will's wedding or Catherine's graduation. How long will he be able to work? And then the realization hit me that I might not be growing old with him the way I'd hoped. The worst part of this phase was not letting him see how terrified and upset I was. I cried in parking lots a lot. My tissues were with me at the grocery store, my work, his work, Yale, the commuter lot of I-95, the bank. Anywhere I could release the fear and anger so it wouldn't affect Bruce. He didn't need to worry about me, as all his energy needed to be focused on a positive "I can live with this" attitude.

The surgery was planned for May 6. We immediately went in to talk with his boss. Bruce had worked for a small manufacturing company in Branford, Connecticut, for twelve years, and we'd been told he was considered part owner. However, there was nothing formal on paper. We told the truth about our situation. We looked for a college intern to help out. The plan was that Bruce would have his surgery and I'd adjust my work hours and do my day job from 7am to 3pm. Then I'd drive over to his job and help out from 3:30pm to 8pm. The intern would fill in where he could. That way the small company would not be affected by his absence.

We didn't want to tell our kids. Our daughter was taking finals at Georgetown and our son was getting ready to leave for a State Department rotation in Guatemala. His fiancé was finishing her Masters at George Washington and they were elbow deep in wedding planning and trying to discuss budget with me. I stalled. My justification was we'd tell them when we knew more.

Was this sporadic or genetic? Bruce and I decided to tell the kids once their exams were done and he was through his first surgery. What's that old saying? When we make plans, God laughs?

Our son came into town the morning of the surgery. We picked him up at the train station, told him our situation, and drove over to the hospital to admit Bruce. The boy takes after his parents. He didn't want to spoil the bride and groom's day and went to the rehearsal dinner that night and the wedding the next day without ever letting on there was an issue.

Bruce's surgery took 12 hours. It was much more extensive than they'd originally thought, and he sacrificed a vocal cord. I was in the waiting room during the surgery. They use these huge monitors so you can see when your loved one was pre-surgery, during the procedure, and when he was in recovery. Bruce's name disappeared around the 7th hour in. I found my courage and asked about his status, but they didn't know.

When his surgeon came walking around the corner I came close to passing out. After seeing me his first words were, "He's alive". The surgery was much more involved than we thought. We're waiting for a thoracic surgeon to help.

Bruce made it through surgery and was in intensive care for ten days. He had another surgery in June, this time a seven-hour procedure to clean out the rest. They took everything on the left side of his neck, which resulted in a chyle leak. He again spent another ten days in the hospital.

On July 4, I even assisted the surgeon in his office as he replaced a drain that was coming out of Bruce's incision. The office was closed and there were no nurses around. The surgeon left his family barbeque to meet us. I've never been able to handle any type of first aid without passing out, but for Bruce I do whatever it takes.

The fix didn't work and he began to look like a bullfrog, all puffed up, so he had another surgery in July to fix the chyle leak. The surgeon met us at the emergency entrance, put Bruce in a wheelchair and took him directly to the surgical suite upstairs without any documentation. This doctor cares and does what it takes whenever anything needs to be done. Bruce was allowed to come home in two days. He wore a neck brace for ten days to stabilize the neck and not disturb the drains. I learned how to do pressure dressings, empty drains, and prepare no-fat meals.

I broke down and finally called my mother for help. This was the beginning of my learning to accept help from others. Mom stayed until mid-August, helping me shop, prepare meals and be my eyes when I couldn't be with Bruce.

The endocrinologist called with good news. "It was sporadic, no mutations." Okay, time for a breath. But being the nervous mom I am, I still made my kids get a calcitonin test so at least we'd have a baseline.

Regarding work, we kept meeting with the business owner and I kept working the two jobs. Bruce tried to go back to work part-time. Mom drove him and reminded the owner he was only to work a couple of hours, after which I'd be in to get him.

August 2013. The end of summer came, and with it, six weeks of radiation, a hurricane, and Bruce being terminated. He called me at work, devastated, and told me his boss just said, "We're a small company and I can't afford to continue things the way they are. I'll give you unemployment, and when you're better let's get together and see where we stand." It was the first time Bruce had been unemployed since he was 14. Bruce had worked for this man for twelve years without vacations or raises, helping grow the business into a successful small company. The owner kept promising bonuses that never materialized. We were told to consider the business part ours, and the owner would deal with the lawyers to work out the details. Guess he did, because he got the company and Bruce got fired.

My immediate response was, "Don't worry about it. Your health is more important. You don't need the stress and you don't need him or that job." We saw a lawyer about the termination and were told companies under 15 employees did not have to abide by federal laws.

Besides, how could Bruce interview for a new job without a voice? I spent that night filling out Social Security Disability forms online. The next night I researched tax codes to see how to access his 401K so we could pay down our debt.

When I found my MTC family, it was such a relief. They held my hand, answered my questions and were always there. It was the support I needed. I could communicate by typing and they wouldn't see me cry. They always knew just what to say to give me the courage and energy to face the next day.

Bruce was exhausted and worn out. In May he weighed 264 pounds, and by August he was down to 184. Most of that weight came off due to the no-fat diet from June to August. The radiation burns were severe. He could barely swallow, and major fatigue set in.

November came and Bruce was partly back on his feet, but he was weak. He had a Gore-Tex implant on November 17 to fix his voice and help him swallow without choking. Surgery was successful with only an overnight stay.

We decided to collect our kids from DC and drive to Hendersonville, North Carolina, and have a family Thanksgiving. We had a lot to be thankful for. Bruce was slowly recovering. Every day he had a little more energy, his mouth was a little less dry, and he could speak and be heard. The blood work was coming back elevated but stable. Social Security Disability came through and our money issues eased a bit. The wedding was planned for March and the bride and groom understood we were not in a position to contribute. I swallowed my pride and called Georgetown University to discuss our financial situation. They revisited my daughter's financial aid package. Again, this was a growing moment for me, as I hate to ask for anything and it's much easier for me to give than to receive.

The wedding day arrived and I once again found myself crying in parking lots, the church, the hotel, and the reception venue. They were tears of gratitude this time, because this was a milestone I didn't think Bruce would achieve. My daughter's graduation came. Another milestone. Our youngest went off on her own to Kansas City. We'd made it to "empty nesters." I remember thinking that MTC has made me value each of these things so much more.

Bruce was feeling better, eating better, and looking better. Okay, we can do this. Get blood drawn every three months and be a nervous wreck. Get the results and breathe again.

Bruce is my house hubby, doing laundry and meals. I work and provide income and insurance. This year sucked, but we reorganized. We didn't panic, we rode the crazy train. We played Whack-a-Mole and we survived. Other people have chronic diseases. I needed to look at this as I would look at diabetes or heart disease. Love him. Be sure every day he knows what he means to me and my life. Make it a priority.

A year from the date of the start of radiation that damn mole showed his head again. Bruce developed Bell's palsy and one half of his face was paralyzed. *Not* cool. We made another round of doctor visits, hoping and praying it wasn't MTC spreading to his brain. Thankfully, scans were clear. I found a cool eye patch to cover and protect the eye that didn't blink. He was my pirate. Then I bought him a unique hand carved cane to help with balance issues. He looked so dapper and interesting.

We continued to monitor his MTC markers, and they were still stable. His facial nerve was regenerating. We were back on firm ground. The next couple of months saw more monitoring of tumor markers, more adjustments of thyroid replacement hormone, more juggling of doctors and medical bills. Now that things seemed a little more normal, I started falling apart, which coincided with my father passing away at the age of 73 from complications of Parkinson's disease. Bruce was there for me, as he always has been.

I couldn't sleep. More nights than not I'd still be up when Bruce woke for a cup of coffee. His sleep patterns had been thrown off. He woke around 2 or 3am for the day. Once he's up, I could sleep a few hours, and then I'd be off to work. One day it dawned on me I couldn't sleep because I felt I needed to make sure he was doing well. He often was in pain and exhausted when he went to bed, so I stayed up to watch over him. When he woke it was his best time of day and I knew he'd be working on his model railroad and finding some enjoyment in his life. So after sharing a cup of coffee it was "safe" for me to grab a few hours of sleep. He always woke me for work with a cup of coffee and it became a cherished time and a new routine.

My family scheduled a memorial for my dad at Thanksgiving. I'm ashamed to admit it, but all I could think was thank God it wasn't Bruce. I'm the oldest of five kids and his passing was hard on each one of us. I just couldn't relate. It worries me that I've stuffed all that emotion down deep. Will it come back and hit me harder later in life? I was so scared and numb thinking it could have been Bruce that I refused to think about what Dad's death meant to me.

January 2013. Bruce had a routine dental appointment that turned into a root canal, then a tooth extraction. But due to the radiation that became a whole new drama of heavy-duty antibiotics and painkillers. Okay, not so bad. Except later that month at the oncologist his white blood count was up. The doctor said it probably had to do with something his body was fighting and we needed to come back the next week and have labs redrawn.

My stomach hit the floor. I immediately Googled this, and I *knew* what she was thinking. We waited a week and went back to do the blood work. Again the results showed an elevated count, but the oncologist was not saying anything. She kept looking at paperwork, and finally said, "I need you to go to Yale and have a bone marrow biopsy."

Bruce told her, "Whatever you need, I'll do."

I said, "You think it might be leukemia?" She just looked at me. I continued, "Let me rephrase that. Do you want to rule out leukemia?"

She slowly answered yes. I started crying in the doctor's office for the first time ever. Bruce didn't want to spend the night in the hospital and I didn't blame him. He asked if she could do it in her office without anesthesia. I admired his strength and courage. It looked like after a painful day we were back whacking that mole.

The oncologist called and confirmed Bruce had chronic myeloid leukemia (CML). We made another appointment to see her. She explained there was great success treating this with a **tyrosine-kinase inhibitor** (TKI) called Gleevec. She went on to explain Bruce would have oral chemotherapy and would be on it the rest of his life. It had some nasty side effects. She wrote the prescription.

Bruce was taking this pretty well. Maybe we were just shell shocked. We drove over to Stop and Shop to fill the prescription and were told our co-pay every month for this drug would be $3,100 dollars! The cost of the drug was $9,000 a month. I was speechless. Here I was standing in the store trying to calculate how much and for how long I could charge this before we went bankrupt. Bruce came up behind me and said, "No. I'm on borrowed time anyway, and I'm not going to die leaving you alone and bankrupt. We'll go home, plan the trip of a lifetime, and when we come home, I'll die."

I turned back to the pharmacist and said, "Okay, that's not going to happen. We can't afford it." The pharmacist came out from around the counter and told me to contact Novartis directly. They might have patient assistant programs for people who couldn't afford their medications.

Another moment of growth. I called, choked out my problem and they were very nice. They told me I needed to provide basically the same information you'd provide for your kids' financial aid for college or for a mortgage. After being thoroughly vetted they decided to foot the bill 100 percent due to our income. I was shocked.

March 2013. Bruce was back on board, doing what it took to live life. He started the TKI in late March. The side effects were not good, but he hung in there. We were scheduled for weekly visits to monitor blood and TSH levels because the leukemia medications don't play nice with the TSH medications. We monitored his diet to control chronic diarrhea and cramping, and avoided the sun. Slowly his body adjusted to the oral chemotherapy and he reached major molecular response. We celebrated that he was stable with both cancers. We also celebrated our daughter-in- law's graduation from law school. We helped them move from DC to NYC.

The National Honor Society of the school where I worked presented me with a check. These high school students said they knew health expenses ate up a lot of income and wanted to help in a small way. These were teenagers who wanted to help an adult in their school system whom they normally didn't have much interaction with. One of them had overheard a teacher asking how my husband was doing, and thought this would be a way to make a difference. I was so humbled by their generosity and graciously accepted their gift.

November 2013. It was the week before Thanksgiving, bringing more monitoring of blood work for both MTC and CML. We were determined to live life to the fullest and were thinking of the coming holiday and family. We got a phone call telling us that calcitonin and CEA were beginning to creep up. Wait and watch. Okay, we knew this might happen. Lots of people's results blip and burp. The oncologist would recheck Bruce's levels in January. She told us to have a wonderful holiday season and she'd see us in January.

January 2014. Tumor markers up again. Bruce had another PET scan. Where previously no MTC metastasis was found, no such luck this time. The scan revealed a mass in his chest and smaller tumor load on his hips.

We just stared at each other. I wasn't talking at all, just sitting in the office while the oncologist and Bruce discussed his situation. They talked about the pros and cons of starting Caprelsa, another TKI. She told us she had searched for someone who had a patient with both these cancers to see how the TKIs would interact. No one knew. Bruce decided to go ahead with the new medication and started Caprelsa in May 2014. While the cost of this drug was $18,000 a month, the pharmacy informed us our monthly co-pay would only be $25.00. Now it seemed we were playing Whack-a-Mole and Monopoly with play money and TKIs.

At first Bruce was monitored weekly with EKGs, blood work and office visits. He controlled the hand and foot rash with bag balm, vasoline, mineral oil and cotton gloves. If he had to do any work with his hands he used padded bicycle gloves to diminish the friction that shredded his fragile skin.

The TKIs were doing their jobs. MTC tumors shrank considerably and the CML was back in major molecular response. The insurance denied the request for a PET scan, as his tumor markers were so low. This made me happy. Bruce had a CT scan instead and continued to show shrinkage and improved blood work.

Life has changed. What would have bothered me before, asking for help and accepting someone's goodwill, or writing all this down for someone to read, doesn't feel so uncomfortable anymore. Everyone has challenges in life. I plan to wake up every morning and live in the day, thankful for Bruce. While I'm busy with his interests, he's doing the same for me. He wakes me every morning with a smiling face and a mug of coffee. Every night when I come in the door there's some yummy concoction coming out of the oven waiting to be served. After 35 years of marriage, it's the little daily things that give us both the courage to face the future, however long that may be.

Here are the answers I've found. How long does he have? He has long enough to feel the love of those around him and know he matters to all of us.

How much suffering will he go through? Can I be strong enough to help him through this? He'll go through a lot of suffering, and by watching him struggle I can find the strength to help him when he needs me.

Will we get through this? Of course we will. We're strong and love each other and took vows to be there for each other. I'm not ready to lose him. And I'll never be ready to lose him. He wasn't supposed to be around for Will's wedding or Catherine's graduation, but he not only celebrated those events but also the birth of our first grandchild. Come this December he and I will celebrate our daughter's wedding.

How long will he be able to work? Between the surgeries, radiation, Bell's palsy, leukemia, and the start of two oral chemotherapies it hasn't been possible for him to work. Thank goodness for Social Security Disability.

What about the realization that I may not be growing old with him the way I counted on? I don't know the answer to this yet. So far I truly feel the life I share with Bruce has gotten a lot dearer and sweeter to me.

Do we have years ahead? Maybe. I value every single day, banking these memories to cherish if I grow old without him.

It's not really the "you have cancer" that took my breath away. It was the fear of the unknown future living with cancer that took my breath away.

Meddie Memoir

By Myrtle L. Young

My cowboy daddy used to say, "What doesn't kill you only makes you stronger."

Another saying was, "It's a long way from your heart, so stop your crying."

I've thought a lot about previous life experiences, family culture and influences, as well as community environment – all of which have had a definite impact on who I am today. What have I learned and experienced that shapes the woman I am today? I don't believe that I've been truly tested to the core, but I do believe I'm determined and resilient. I am thankful that I've been blessed with wonderful family and lifelong friends that enrich my life daily, always overshadowing the darkest days. A fulfilling career in the world of juvenile court services showed me just how rich I was to have those dozens upon dozens of individuals helping to shape my life. But genetics? I never could have dreamed the role that this untold territory of my genes would play.

Now my genes were not a part of me that I suspected would ever be the "problem child" as I grew into adulthood. I always hung on to the thought that having "good" genes is what's going to get me through all the "bad" I've subjected my body to over the years. Not unusual to hear me throw out, "longevity runs in my family." My maternal grandpa lived to be 102, my grandmother, lived to be 93 and my mother lived to be over 92, as did three of her siblings. So no matter how much I lived trying to fill every breathing moment being productive, worked long hours and distances in an exciting but demanding / stress-filled job, chose to not eat healthily, over indulged with alcohol as a self-medicating solution to any problem or as an excuse to celebrate, I kind of figured I would fade into the sunset as the glorious dame on the western frontier. I wasn't so egocentric to think I'd live forever, but well... at least I'd probably live for a very long time, because I had darn good genes! I pretty much thought I was invincible.

My first experience with medullary thyroid cancer (MTC) didn't start with me. When one of my dearest friends, Cindy (who I first met in my new grown up world in post college days and who was always by my side for those carefree 20's and 30's decades) called me years later to inform me she woke up one morning and couldn't get out of bed, little did I know that I would later become all too familiar with this devastating disease. I recall that with all good intentions, I would repeatedly ask her why this thyroid cancer couldn't be contained, she finally told me in an exasperating explanation, "You don't understand. What I have is a very rare type of thyroid cancer." I can't even remember her telling me the name of the cancer. Too few years passed before I lost her, visiting her at her new home in Florida several times as she deteriorated before my very eyes.

A couple of years later when I accidently discovered that I had a nodule within my thyroid after undergoing an employer provided preventive carotid artery scan, I began an extensive journey just to find out what it was. Never was I really encouraged to proactively get to the bottom of what this nodule was except for the ultrasound technician that fateful day in 2007. I wish I could find him to hug his neck and thank him. But even as curious and determined as I was, I could never fathom that someday I would be reliving the same diagnosis that Cindy had been given. For many years, my surgeon's words on the phone reverberated back, "Myrtle, I'm surprised to tell you that your pathology report reflects that you have this very rare cancer."

This call came after an anxious wait for the pathology report from my first incomplete surgery. The surgeon made the decision to remove only half of my thyroid to check out what he was convinced was what he called "the easy cancer". I really can't remember what else he said that day other than wanting to set me up for a second surgery to remove the other half of my thyroid. All I can remember is quietly going outside that spring day to sit in my garden, staring into space. Those haunting words kept coming back to me from years back, "…you don't understand, I have this very rare cancer." The reality finally hit. I have the same cancer that took the life of my very dear friend, Cindy. I continued to sit there stunned for hours.

I should have known the hurdles to come. After doing a fast and furious research on the internet between that date of diagnosis and the second scheduled surgery, I quickly learned a simple thyroid removal would not suffice as this was a disease that traveled microscopically very early on, that it was slow growing in many cases, but, "the cat is more than likely out of the bag" being the most common scenario. I remember reading from a renowned expert in a published paper that the surgeons who say they can tell with the naked eye that they got it all are most likely sadly mistaken. As I called my primary physician, my endocrinologist who referred me to this particular surgeon, and my family, I was met with a myriad of opinions. My primary physician listened to a direct explanation from the surgeon who convinced her that this was more than likely contained and it might not be in my best interest to do a full neck dissection. When I called my endo, he told me in a very self-assured way, well of course you're going to have a full neck dissection that was the proper protocol. However, he never did call the surgeon to whom he referred me in order to convey my concern or to ascertain that was indeed the protocol that would be followed. Hours before my second surgery, I finally received a message from my surgeon assuring me that he would be seeing me the next day and, "Not to worry. AND NO, you don't need a neck dissection."

When I was in pre-op for the second surgery, the surgeon came in to assure me that he would be ordering RAI for me, just to make extra sure the cancer would not return. It was then I knew I had a doctor who knew less about this cancer than I did. Lying there telling him that I had researched this cancer and that I understood that RAI didn't apply to MTC, he patted me on the shoulder and told me I read too much on the internet. I passively succumbed to the second surgery, still yet to have any lymph nodes removed to determine if there was any spread, although my cancerous nodule was close to 1.4 cm, the "cat's probably out of the bag" size.

My quest to stay one step ahead of this beast that had killed my friend, by learning all I could, began in earnest. The next hurdle came from my endocrinologist. He told me, after doing a test to rule out pheochromocytomas, that I was sporadic. Since my children were adopted, I didn't need genetic testing. When I asked about my siblings and the potential impact on them if I had inherited this disease, he told me it was very expensive and not necessary. My search for a second opinion began.

It was increasingly clear that genetic testing was one step I needed to take to better understand not only my situation but that of my three full siblings, and half-sister. But selfishly, I had already heard Dr. Gagel at a ThyCa conference speak to a mutation that even sporadic patients had, which if identified, could better predict how aggressive a person's MTC might be. I knew little to nothing of autosomal vs somatic, but just knew it might be an important component. The struggle to get genetic testing took another year but proved to be worth it. I discovered that I did have a rare deviant, k666n, with unknown significance. My mother, 90 years old at the time, was the carrier. The fact that my mother was still living, swayed and blinded many of my family and doctors, even at the Arizona Cancer Center. I was told by the new "second opinion" guy that I was still more than likely sporadic. Apparently, he never read my file after genetic testing, nor acknowledged my mother tested positive until I asked him how could I be considered sporadic if my mother was a carrier. He mumbled some answer that convinced me it was a fluke in nature. Via our internet group and ThyCa conferences, my newfound meddie friends kept me focused on getting a clearer answer from Dr. Cote at MD Anderson, who encouraged me to come back home and advocate for my siblings to be tested. Another two years had already passed since I had discovered I carried this rare deviant variant. There was huge skepticism (or denial?) by my siblings, except for one that had gone to her own doctor to ask for genetic testing. Heck, *she* got the testing before *mine* was ever approved. When hers turned out to be negative for this mutation, I believe my other siblings began to feel bullet proof. Here our mother was still alive, our one sister was negative and, well, look at Myrtle, she looked perfectly fine. After months and years of being made to feel that I was simply scaring the heck out of my siblings, I can thankfully report that my two other siblings, although testing positive for the K666N mutation, have now been able to seek medical screening for MTC. My oldest sister had surgery in 2014 and her thyroid tested positive for MTC. My younger brother, after having moved out of the country, has finally been approved for medical treatment in Sweden and is seeing a specialist for determination of nodules within his thyroid. Two of their children have thus far tested positive for this mutation. More testing of others will follow. I find no solace that searching out genetic testing proved that my siblings and their children are impacted by medullary cancer. But I do feel a great sense of relief that our family is no longer burying their heads in the sand.

My story doesn't lead me down the path of advanced Medullary Cancer yet. But watching and tracking lesions on my liver and ilium has taken me into another dark world of wondering when the other shoe will drop. Although that term might be overused, it truly applies to those of us who have shown great labs, stable scans, and none of the late stage symptoms of MTC. What is causing that swollen lump in my neck? What is the reason for any one thing going wrong? From a simple cold, to aching joints, to unexplained punches below my ribcage. I wonder. I worry. Is my Medullary Cancer on the march? I cannot totally let go of these irrational fears. But as I grow older and have learned to live in a neighborly fashion with this disease, I find myself occupied with the accumulation of other ills that shove MTC to the background, like new neighbors on the block. A diagnosis of Rheumatoid Arthritis is more than a distraction, it is in direct competition for my daily attention.

MTC has changed my life forever. To be perfectly clear, I don't trust it one bit. I liken it to a forbe found in the Arizona desert called 'cat-claw'. I try to prune back its wild and unruly branches, but just as I'm about to throw off the branch, it catches me with its tiny hooked thorns.

I have never wondered "why me?" Why other friends who were diagnosed with breast cancer, pancreatic cancer, and colon cancer? The fact of the matter is, I've been enriched by this fate of genetics, this 50/50 toss of the coin. The compassion and sense of brotherhood and sisterhood I feel for my fellow "meddies' is now fully embedded into my heart and soul. This camaraderie I feel towards those I've met and those I've never met outside this virtual world of ours, is a kinship.

The Insidious Lump

By Karen Dewey

One day, feeling fine and really quite fit ...Yes, one day last July I found a lump that changed my life, and the lives of those who love me, forever.

I found a lump. "What could it be?"
My physio friend said, "Wait and see."
It may go down, but if it stays or grows,
Go to your GP, the "One who knows."

It stayed the same for a week or two.
In the back of my mind, I think I knew.
I Googled cancer tumour in neck.
No mindful peace, I think I'll check!

My GP didn't mess around.
Said, "To be safe, an ultrasound."
I'll mark it "urgent," just in case.
Wait for results, then we'll touch base.

Two days later an urgent call:
"Come in quickly!" No info at all.
I called my mum. "I'm going to die."
Explained to her, and started to cry.

They'd taken a sample, an FNA.
I'd been given no explanation that day.
The sample was blood, nothing else had been found.
But lymph nodes were oval, and this one was round.

I had the test repeated again.
This time by a gun, to ascertain
Exactly what this lump could be.
Very distressing the wait would be.

"Meddies" have given this worry a name.
Welcome aboard the anxiety train!
I knew in my heart the result would be bad.
I didn't want to make my family sad.

Already lost dad, son Jon, 18, in a crash
And Julian, my nephew, in a motorbike smash.
My family couldn't take any more.
We'd already all been cut to the core.

The hospital called. I've got thyroid cancer.
"Which one?" I asked, and waited for the answer.
"Medullary, and it is very rare."
At least not anaplastic, that was my scare!

I wanted to know and asked, "Can it be treated?"
The lady said, "Yes", but first hesitated.
I'd mentally prepared myself to die.
Beside my son I would surely lie.

I saw my consultant, an ENT.
After an MRI scan, he would admit me
To be cut ear to ear. The scar, it would heal.
He'd remove thyroid and nodes and make a good seal!

I dreaded the day, but to hinder this thing
Was my only objective, more time would it bring.
The staples were many, I looked like a freak.
My neck was so stiff, and I felt very weak.

I told my consultant that I wish I had died.
My night had been sleepless. "I hate it," I cried.
Things just got worse. I was hypocalcemic.
My body in spasm, I'd never felt so sick.

I had drains from my neck, dripping chyle on my nightdress,
And nurses all hours there to help clean up the mess.
I felt dirty and ugly, blood dried in my hair.
No make-up or shower, but my family was there.

To help me and love me, to see me right through,
So I had to get better, 'cos I loved them, too.
I go for a massage, my neck needs this care.
To loosen the tendons and muscles in there.

I ate veggies and fruit, the diet was a bore.
I didn't think I could take any more!
At last I could leave, would I ever be well?
CEA and calcitonin doubling times would tell.

I've two spots on my lung, I hope they won't grow.
Will be checked for changes. I will go with the flow.
This cancer can spread to kidneys and liver.
The thought of this prognosis makes me shiver.

Five months down the line I do have a life.
Had a wonderful holiday, and will soon be a wife.
I know what's important, not material things.
Don't take life for granted, accept what it brings.

Your life can be taken, without any warning.
Who knows if you'll even wake up in the morning?
Our families are precious, the last thing I'll say
Is to cherish and love them. . . LIVE LIFE FOR THE DAY!!

Waiting For The Waterfall

By ToniAnne Murray

I started feeling neck pain in early 2009. It was a deep sore throat pain, so I went to my primary physician, who kept telling me it was allergies. It didn't go away as the seasons changed, and in 2010 I went to an ENT who examined me with a scope and could not find a reason for my throat pain. It had increased to daily throbbing.

Frustrated beyond belief, the next month I went to my primary physician and sat in his office and demanded that he do an ultrasound of my neck. The technician did the exam and my primary physician came in and told me they found a 2.1cm vascular nodule in the left node of the thyroid.

I returned with these results to my ENT for follow-up. The ENT did a fine needle aspiration. The results were that the mass was most likely papillary thyroid cancer, and the results would probably be good once he removed my thyroid.

My ENT sent the fine need aspiration and ultrasound results to Baptist Hospital, who reviewed the information and reported the fine need aspiration was uncertain and the pathologist at Baptist Hospital thought it was most like papillary carcinoma, although the possibility of MTC was mentioned. On December 6, 2010, my ENT scheduled my thyroid removal on his belief that it was papillary. Upon removal of my thyroid the pathology report showed a 2.5 x 1.3 x 1.0cm medullary carcinoma. There was an extension into perithyroidal fat that was called minimal and the surgery margins were positive. Three of the five left central compartment nodes were positive for MTC.

Prior to surgery, my ENT did not perform a CEA or calcitonin blood test because he was going on the belief that it was papillary. Two days after surgery I returned to my ENT for a follow-up and he then performed a CEA and calcitonin blood test. The results showed CEA was 3.42 and calcitonin was less than two.

Due to the finding of MTC and having never heard of this type of cancer I went to Duke University Hospital. Duke reviewed all the scans, ultrasounds and tissues and also performed more neck ultrasounds and PET scans. Upon review by Duke it was found that I had a 1.9 cm left level IV lymph node. PET scan was clean. Excisional biopsy of the left level IV was carried out on February 28, 2011, and the frozen sections were negative so the procedure was ended. The surgeon declared me "cured" and sent me home.

Three days later the surgeon called me and told me that the surgical specimen showed that two of the seven lymph nodes he removed were positive for MTC and wanted me to return immediately for a "total neck dissection."

At this point I was floored and confused and researched MTC. I found I was in the wrong place, as none of the doctors who had examined me, performed surgery on me, and reviewed pathological results really had any concept or understanding of this disease.

Researching the Web I found the Facebook thyroid group and ThyCA.org and learned of Dr. Ball at Johns Hopkins University Hospital.

All my information was sent and Dr. Ball accepted me as an MTC patient. I began seeing him on September 11, 2011.

I presently have three 1cm lymph nodes in level IV. One is positive for MTC and another central node is being watched. I follow with him on a six-month basis, with three to six-month blood work to watch my CEA and calcitonin.

Since the surgery, my calcitonin has doubled every six months. I met with Dr. Ball's surgeon at Johns Hopkins, and he was extremely hesitant to do surgery because of the prior two surgeries. The risks outweighed the possible results at this point.

So here I stand and wait for this disease to progress. People who find I have incurable cancer do a double take and actually say, "but you look so good." All of this just thrusts me deeper into denial. At the time of my diagnosis my mother suffered vascular strokes with dementia, and I spent the last three years taking care of her until her death in December 2014.

I keep my appointments with Dr. Ball. I do what I have to do to take care of myself, but I have put my acceptance of my own cancer on the proverbial back burner. My own mother was not even aware of my cancer at the time of her passing. Denial has become my best friend, my safety net, my answer.

I've tried therapy twice, but the therapist did not even know of MTC. I felt she could not understand what I was going through. Her advice was to write my feelings on a balloon and just let it go. Needless to say, therapy session three didn't happen.

My OB/Gyn had not ever heard of MTC when I went to her for my appointments. Denial can be a blessing and a curse, but the lack of knowledge in the medical profession is frustrating, and I feel I need to check every prescription and procedure with Dr. Ball so as to not interfere with the care he is providing.

I feel blessed that my cancer has not progressed in the past four years to the point of further surgery or metastasis to other parts of my body (that I'm aware of). I have cried over the progression of this disease and loss of the friends I met through the Facebook and ThyCA.org sites. The kinship I feel is my blessing and my grief. Those who read this and have this cancer, or have someone close to them with it will understand. Those who don't, won't.

I feel like I live on a log in the middle of a river, waiting for it to hit the waterfall. I don't know how long the river is, when I will reach the waterfall, what obstructions I may face down the river, so I float and live and wait.

My name is ToniAnne Murray and I am a Medullary cancer fighter and survivor.

I Realize How Short Life Can Be

By Becky Post

Each year I like to set some goals and resolutions. I started putting my goals in place for 2013 early in December 2012. I was set on returning to school to finish my degree by the end of summer 2013. I also wanted to make some fitness goals to help challenge me in 2013.

I'm a planner. I like to plan things out in detail. When there's not a plan in place it makes me CRAZY! When my little sister would come spend the summer I'd have an itinerary put together for the whole summer. My husband, Art, now asks for an itinerary when we go on vacation. It's very rare when I'm not planning something in life.

Well, sometimes things happen in life, and no matter how much planning I do, my plans get thrown to the side. 2013 has already been turned upside down. In December I went to the doctor for some stomach issues. She found a lump on my thyroid. Totally not something I knew about or even had gone to see her about. The doctor ordered an ultrasound of my thyroid. I fell asleep during the procedure. The tech had to wake me up to move my neck so they could finish the ultrasound. The results showed my thyroid had a large growth on it, so an MRI was ordered.

I take after my dad completely in the sleep department. I had ear plugs and was strapped down for the MRI, but I fell asleep in that nosy machine. The tech had to wake me up to see if I was okay. I was told I'd have my results back in 2-3 business days. The next morning my doctor called with the results. She wanted to send me for a thyroid biopsy. I left work immediately and went to get the biopsy.

The doctor bypassed an endocrinologist and sent me directly to a head and neck surgeon. I had a biopsy of my thyroid, and this time I did not fall asleep. Two days later the doctor called stating they weren't sure if I had thyroid cancer or just an extremely under-active thyroid. My right thyroid was enlarged, but the left side was extremely enlarged. My left thyroid went down my throat and reached my breastbone. It was also pushing on my windpipe. The doctor scheduled surgery and asked me to come in the next day for another biopsy of my lymph node.

The next appointment and biopsy took a turn I never thought I would face. The doctor talked about other possibilities besides thyroid cancer. They were concerned I could possibly have lymphoma, based on the size of my lymph nodes. The biopsy was more extensive and we'd have to wait for the results to find out exactly what the next steps would be.

The biopsy came back thyroid cancer. However, the doctors were still concerned about lymphoma. They said they'd pull out a lymph node to test during surgery, and if it was lymphoma they'd remove my thyroid and close me up pending additional treatment. If it was thyroid cancer they'd remove my thyroid and all the lymph nodes.

I was trying to deal with classes and health issues, and then I got a terrible respiratory infection. I contacted my counselor at school and ended up dropping all my classes. There was no way I could keep up with school and deal with surgery or cancer treatments.

My plans for 2013 were completely turned upside down with just one phone call. I think the hardest part was telling my family. Making those phone calls to my parents to deliver test results and tell them it was cancer were the worst to make. One of my grandmas called, very concerned. I told her it was all going to be just fine and she shouldn't worry. At the end of the call she said, "You've calmed me right down and I was supposed to be calming you down." The other grandma offered to come to California to help take care of me, but she couldn't drive me around unless I was able to give her very clear directions.

I took pictures from the morning I left my house for surgery until a week later. I actually took pictures almost every day. I'd told myself I'd let myself cry when I saw my scar and I wouldn't cry anymore. But I didn't cry when I saw my incision. I was actually relieved to see the doctor had cut much lower than she'd originally told me. I was to have been cut in the middle of my neck; instead she cut me around the base of my neck. The incision is not that bad, and it's healing very nicely.

Pre-op was probably my favorite part of the course, since there was no pain involved. They gave me a gown with places they could insert a tube to blow in hot air. The tube was attached to the gown around my thigh, and I had a controller for how warm I wanted the air. This machine was used in both pre-op and in the operating room. It was *heaven*! I seriously want one of those machines for home. I joked around the entire hour before surgery with my fabulous nurse, Gloria.

I kept my sense of humor until I had to kiss Art good bye. That was the first time I felt scared. I was more scared for him, because I knew the next 8-10 hours would be very hard. I had the easiest part. The worst part was for the family.

As we walked to the OR I asked the nurse how in the world she could work back there. It was freezing. Seriously, it was like an ice box. I walked into the OR and said to my doctor, "I'm walking in to this room and I'll walk out, right?" She said they'd give me a break and take me out a little easier. The doctor assured me I'd be just fine and recover great because I had the best attitude through the whole process. I met everyone in the OR, talked to them, joked with them, lay on the bed, and started to get some drugs. The doctors did an overview of everything by reading patient name, medical record number, procedure, and other stuff I can't remember anymore. It was honestly surreal to listen to them. Even as I lay on the table I couldn't believe I was the one lying there for surgery.

When I woke up from surgery I was *pissed*! Why in the world were they waking me up *already*? I had finally started to get some great rest and these people were waking me up. I asked, "What time is it?" They said, "7:00 p.m." That was my cue everything was just fine and I didn't need to worry about lymphoma. If the surgery had been shorter, then I had lymphoma.

I went back to sleep. I remember waking up on and off, and the first memory I had was of my doctor sitting across the room from me at a desk. I guess that was while I was in the ICU. I remember them taking blood and an x-ray. They moved me to a room, and then, *bam*! I was smacked in the face with *pain*.

The pain that Friday night was *horrific*! Someone brought me a dinner, broth in a bowl with a spoon. Thinking back, this cracks me up. I couldn't even move, but I was supposed to eat broth with a spoon?

It didn't matter how much pain medication they gave me, nothing helped. I remember lying in bed that night as I dozed on and off, thinking I'd never be able to move again. My shoulders, back and neck were *super* sore. In fact, I couldn't move my shoulders at all. The nurse helped by putting a pillow behind my back. My overnight nurse, Sarah, was simply amazing! She'd make sure I wasn't in pain; bringing me pain medications before I had to ask for them, and helping me drink some chicken broth. This woman even gave me a sponge bath.

Art came to the hospital around 9:30 a.m. on Saturday. It had been the longest 12 hours without him. At some point I realized I had on a different hospital gown. I pulled on my gown and said, "Wait a minute. Someone saw me *naked* because I'm changed." We just started laughing.

My daytime nurse, Belinda, was amazing! She helped move me, so I had some relief. I was a little concerned I'd get bed sores. I kept asking people to help me move. She helped me eat my liquid breakfast and made sure I was comfortable. I was able to get out of bed around lunchtime to sit in a chair. I sat up while my friend Cindy visited. One of my first texts on Saturday was to Cindy, asking her to bring me a hair tie. I couldn't find mine and my hair was making me crazy. When she got there I asked her to put my hair up for me because I couldn't move my arms above my shoulders. My pastor and his wife came to visit me. They were super sweet during this whole thing. My pastor had come to the hospital the morning of surgery and sat with us for a little while. Then he prayed with us prior to surgery.

Different people would come in to check on how I was doing. Every time a new person came in they'd comment on the fact that I was wearing makeup. I went one day without make up and that was enough. I needed to get back into the swing of things, and I refused to look like I was sicker than I was. Sunday night was the best night of sleep I got in the hospital.

When my drains were removed on Monday, one side hurt horrifically. I screamed as they pulled it out. The doctor said part of it must have been wrapped around something up inside my neck and that's why it hurt so badly. When he pulled it out stuff went flying on the bed and on the doctor's face, and his arms. He walked out of the room. I told Cindy I could feel something wet, but I couldn't feel anything else. All of a sudden we saw a big clot of stuff that looked like a worm. I yelled, "Don't touch it! Get the doctor." I was worried Cindy would be grossed out. Cindy found the doctor washing his face. He said part of it might have just been stuck inside.

The doctor came back about 20-30 minutes later and said my doctor told him to remove the other drain. Oh, Lord, I was scared. Cindy held my hand again as I braced for pain, but there wasn't any. The drain just slid right out and it was no big deal. The doctor said that was normally how they should come out.

Monday night I came home from the hospital. I was exhausted. I sat on the couch and couldn't move. Art ran to the store for pudding, as I'd been eating pudding with my pain pills and wanted some that night. When he came back I was sitting there, bawling. I was scared to be home because of the pain and being super tired. I didn't like how swollen my neck was. I just felt awful. On and off the entire night I would just start crying. All the emotions were finally hitting me like a train. Needless to say, I didn't sleep very well.

Tuesday was my first full day home. The swelling started to go down a little and my neck was healing. Wednesday the swelling went down some more. Wednesday we met with the endocrinologist and went over a lot of information. Each time I left the doctor I'd feel I was on overload. I was to meet with her again once the pathology report came back and we'd know what the next steps would be.

My neck was so swollen at one point I looked like Fat Bastard from Austin Powers. When I walked and talked my neck would jiggle. Ugh! The swollen neck has been the worst part for me. I knew I'd have some swelling, but not the amount I did have.

I'd been able to reduce my pain pills quite a bit since I'd come home from the hospital. Some days I experienced more pain than other days. Saturday was a really rough pain day. All the other days the pain had felt more like an ache. It would start off like a toothache and then spread all the way around my chest. Saturday the pain came on like a shooting sharp pain. I had to increase the pain medications so I could sleep for the night.

I knew the recovery would be hard. I couldn't have imagined in 100 years how rough it would be to wake up from surgery. I had morphine last year when I ended up in the ER, and it was amazing. The first day it did nothing. Luckily, once I was able to get past the first night I was able to tolerate the pain better each day. I had to learn the difference between pain and just being sore.

I am now two and one half years since being diagnosed with MTC. I wasn't able stay pregnant prior to having my thyroid removed. We had eight miscarriages. It was a struggle trying to have a family. I kept saying something was wrong, but the doctors would tell me everything was normal. One year after surgery I got pregnant and stayed pregnant. In September 2014 I delivered my little miracle, George.

I find it is harder to deal with cancer now that I'm a mother. Getting those test results are even harder when they're bad. I think I appreciate motherhood so much more because I realize just how short life can be!

I Would Love To Think This Was Over

By Elba Rosa Rodriguez

After a year of feeling sick, having difficulty swallowing, and not knowing what was wrong, I went to see a doctor. The ENT diagnosed Medullary Thyroid Cancer, an illness I had never heard of before.

I was 59, dreaming about my retirement from the judiciary department with a nice pension to be used to travel around the world, after so many years of study and hard work.

After the news, the surgery was quickly scheduled and in December 2007, a new life began.

In April 2008, I was admitted at MD Anderson and immediately another surgery was performed, this time in my head, on the left temporal area.

I had to quit my job, and the journey continued. To mention all the pains, agonies, depression, mood changes, and so forth that I suffered, would be to needlessly remind all of the members of the Facebook MTC group what they have had to live through, too.

I therefore choose to tell you how great my experiences have been with the medical expertise at MD Anderson. The people there have become a part of my life, the doctors, the nurses and everybody who takes care of me during my frequent trips from San Juan to Houston.

Early in January 2013, I had a recurrence with my MTC, and that was the beginning of the chemotherapy pill, Caprelsa. The effects of the medication were so many and so bad that many times I thought that I didn't know which was worse, the remedy or the cancer. But I remained on the drug.

My faith was the biggest support. I have held the cross as my safeguard during the whole process and no matter what, I was always sure that Jesus was on my side. I knew that I would get through all this because in my mind, there was HIM with much more suffering than I have ever known.

As of today, after two years in Caprelsa, my calcitonin is 13 and I enjoy the best time since the beginning of all of this. During this time I have been trying to improve my body's condition, especially my muscles and the level of pain. The Internet support group has been a great help; people with the same condition as I have are always there to help each other.

I know this is not the end of the story but it helps a lot to know that after all this nightmare, there is hope. I have learned a lot with this condition. It also helps me to feel like I have some control, to understand the medical terms and to be part of my own treatment.

I know I am talking in past tense, I would love to think this is over, I know that is not the case, nevertheless I am grateful for all the good experiences and because I am a much better human being after this infamous MTC.

I hope that in the near future this will be just a bad memory.

Carpe Diem!

By Patty Dabrowski

"I feel a lump", was the first thing I heard from my PCP. I just thought I was tired and gaining weight because of menopause. I knew I had a sluggish thyroid because a naturalist I had been seeing indicated my thyroid was "weak". After enough time had passed, I knew I had to get to my Doctor to rule out anything more serious. Doctor to surgeon for a biopsy. My surgeon told me regardless of the biopsy, I had to have my thyroid removed. In the back of my head I remember wondering "why?" Can't you just remove the tumor? After the first blood work came back positive for cancer, he ordered that "one last blood test" to rule out the more serious of the cancers and then my phone rang with the dreaded news that I was positive for MTC. You've all had the same experience. I have something called Medullary Thyroid Cancer. It's incurable and clearly I am going to die. Probably the worst thing I've ever experienced is being told I have cancer. My husband wasn't home, he had just left for Georgia for a month long engineering training school for his job as a railroad engineer. I have a wonderful network of friends that all stepped up and filled the void of him being gone and to make sure I stayed intact. Can I wait for him to get home or does he need to leave the class? "We can wait but not too long", was my surgeon's response. That agonizingly long 30 days was horrible as it just consumed me with ongoing thoughts of having cancer. The more I read on the Internet the more frightened I became. "Incurable" is just not a word that I was expecting to hear. I have an incurable cancer. My doctor was a wonderful man and was very straight forward. He told me the cure was the surgery, but I don't think it ever registered with me. Again, the more I read, the more scared I became, until my doctor finally told me to stop. I found the thyca.org website and stuck to that, and then I just stopped looking.

By the time my husband came home we had 3 days left before my surgery. We went to the park, we ate out, and we went to church, where we got anointed by my priest. At that moment, all became calm in my world. I'd done what I could do and it was in God's hands. Frightened beyond my wildest dreams, I went into surgery. The surgery went well, no complications. I woke up with 3 drainage tubes and a massively huge headache (side effects of anesthesia) and a massively huge bandage. I remember them telling me of the possibility of having to cut my sternum muscle and that I might lose a facial muscle which would prohibit me from smiling. When I woke up, I moved my cheek and moved my shoulder, and they both worked! Total thyroidectomy, 76 lymph nodes, 1 salvia gland and some neck tissue. A week later I got my drain tubes removed and the results were in, no sign of the disease noted in any nodes. Praise Jesus what a wonderful thing to hear! I was Stage 2, Sporadic.

When I think back to that time and the stress not only on me but also on my husband, family and my dear friends, I am grateful for my outcome. The residuals from the surgery are just a mere fraction of what it could have been. I pray for those who haven't been as lucky and hope for that cure for those much sicker.

Live life to the fullest and never take anything for granted. Carpe Diem!

Grateful And Lucky

By Marion Sintenie

My story began in early September 2011. It was the first weekend of September and the center of the city was packed with people. This weekend all the old monumental and cultural buildings were a stage for dozens of choirs showing their skills and progress in their 20-minute performances.

Being a singer in a small female choir performing on Sunday, I chose a few performances of other choirs to attend on this Saturday. The choir my sister was singing in (always a pleasure), the choir my mother was singing in (a large choir of more than 60 people, average age 68), and a choir I had been singing in for quite some years, were all on the agenda.

Afterwards I met with some of the choir members and went out for a drink on one of the terraces. Next thing I knew I was looking at my toes in my summer shoes, realizing I was lying down. Slowly my awareness grew. I was lying in an ambulance and a nurse was trying to get me to answer her questions. Behind my head I heard a familiar voice, belonging to the conductor of the choir. She knew me very well and was the one who suggested calling emergency services, remembering that I had had mini strokes years earlier.

Because that was what was going on. I was having a stroke and was on my way to hospital. What a weird and blurry day that was! I remember being in the emergency room, hearing a lot of people and flashes of conversations, going for a scan of my head, being there for hours. My husband arriving, very scared, me trying to calm him with "they're just keeping me for observation." Still trying to get things organized, calling some of the people in my choir with whom I was to perform the next day and apologizing for being in hospital, making sure my husband was taking my conductor friend home and bringing me an overnight bag. I remember being admitted in a stroke unit, being the only one in a four-person room, having my husband and son visiting me in the evening, feeling their fear and me trying to belittle the situation that got really bad after they left.

I tried walking to the bathroom when all of a sudden my left leg no longer supported me. It scared the daylight out of me! In no time the nurses had me back in my bed and made sure I understood I was not allowed to try getting out of my bed on my own.

In the days to follow it became clear I had had a stroke in the right hemisphere of the brain, causing some trouble in the left side of my body. My left lower leg didn't respond to my commands to move and my left forearm decided to do things in its own manner and in its own time.

In the days to follow they had me tested in several ways, trying to find what caused this stroke. I had to learn to walk, in the beginning behind a walker and later on with crutches. I was sent home after 12 days and entered an outpatient rehabilitation program.

When I had a follow-up appointment with my neurologist three weeks later, he told me that the ultrasound of my neck arteries showed a nodule on the left side of my thyroid, and he referred me to an endocrinologist. The doctors kept reassuring me that more than 95 percent of these nodules turn out to be benign. A fine needle aspiration was scheduled, but they did not get enough cells on the first attempt. That was a strange experience, having someone poking my neck again trying to harvest enough material to satisfy the lab assistant.

I was not aware that this would be the first of many more waiting-for-results-days. In the end the results turned out to be inconclusive. Trying to get a grip on things, I searched the Internet for information about thyroid cancer. I was pretty sure that this was not a benign lump, even though the odds of it being malignant were very small. Again, I found myself reassuring my loved ones and family that everything would be fine and that they did not need to worry. Not knowing if this nodule was benign or malignant caused a nervous feeling that I tried to bury by training very hard in my rehabilitation program.

I was still unable to drive myself and was very dependent on other people. Every day someone from work would come over to pick me up from home, take me to the office and back home again. I was not happy with this situation, and it motivated me to work hard to regain my freedom and independence.

A week before Christmas I had the left lobe of my thyroid removed in a diagnostic surgery and went home the next day. Ten days later, at an appointment for removing the stitches, I learned there was a 3.5cm-sized tumor on the removed half of my thyroid. They thought it contained Medullary Thyroid Cancer (MTC). Because of the rarity of this cancer they sent the removed part of my thyroid to another university hospital for a second opinion.

A few days later I had my exit appointment with the rehabilitation doctor who told me I was allowed to drive again. Yeah!

On Monday the 2nd of January 2012, I received a phone call from my surgeon, telling me that the other pathologist confirmed the MTC diagnosis. He set up an appointment with an endocrinologist for all kinds of tests such as blood, urine, and CT scans. This period felt like I had nothing to do with what was happening, as if it was some kind of play I was watching.

After all the tests, my surgeon explained that he was referring me to a colleague of his in a specialized medical center which was very experienced in performing surgeries in advanced thyroid cancer and re-surgeries in the head and neck area. So I met with the professor in February and agreed on surgery two weeks later to remove the other half of my thyroid.

Although I was pretty informed about the surgery, I was not prepared for what was to come. In an almost eight-hour surgery the rest of my thyroid was removed and a central and left-sided neck dissection was performed to remove the lymph tissue. After three nights I was released from hospital. The wound was healing pretty well and I felt optimistic about recovery. Because my left shoulder was very swollen, the surgeon drained it during my follow-up appointment. That felt very relieving. Another big relief was hearing that no metastases were found in the removed lymph tissue.

What I was not prepared for was another surgery three weeks later to remove a seroma that got infected. Or the time this all took to recover, or adjusting to the correct dose of replacement hormone. Or having issues with lymphedema and limitations in the range of motion of my neck, resulting in being dependent on others again because I was not able to drive my car. It took me almost six months to regain enough motion in my neck to be comfortably able to drive again.

This cancer and its treatment are sure not a walk in the park. The treatments by the lymphedema therapist, the massages of the scar tissue, the pain in neck and shoulder and the anxiousness after every blood draw. Even after three years, I still need the treatments and massages. I am doing all the daily exercises to keep the range of motion in my left arm and shoulder, and using medication and doing meditation to help with the stiffness and pain in my neck.

But also the way other people treat me, telling me I look great and that they could barely see the scar, or their disbelief when I explain that most evenings I am not able to do anything because I'm exhausted after a day at work and doing the basic housekeeping chores are things I had to learn to deal with. Sometimes it still hurts.

At the same time this journey has brought me so many good things! I met wonderful people, in real life as well as on line in a Facebook support group. Some friends grew closer. I have had the most profound conversations with people.

In the end I'm a lucky girl. My calcitonin is undetectable, my CEA is in the normal range, and I'm able to live a pretty normal life. I'm living with the love of my life and our son.

This has been a journey to reconnect with my inner self, my true being. I really discovered my strength inside and the flexibility to bounce back and move forward.

I feel very grateful and lucky.

A Lightbulb Moment

By Kristin MacFarland

So, last night and this morning I had some sort of slap in your face type of moment. Call it a realization, awareness, a light bulb going off or what have you. I realized that I've let this cancer be in the forefront of my life for too long now. I didn't even realize I was doing this so much and how much I have been letting it control me in many ways when it comes to my mind and my life. Yes, let's be blunt, I have a pretty shitty cancer and in all honesty it can really suck, but you know what... life goes on. I can *not* let this ludicrous, asshole of a disease define me. Nothing will define me but myself. *I* decide who I want to be, what I want to accomplish in life, where I want to go, and so many other things...not this cancer.

Too often, I have let it make me feel irrelevant, down, lonely and lost. I use it at times as a crutch. Yes, those days I honestly probably didn't feel that great...but you know what...you get up...you keep moving...you breathe and lift your head as high as you can those days. You are alive, you're still here...you're lucky, you're blessed. So I think to myself, "Self, stop bitching, stop complaining, and stop letting this define you!" People have life and situations so much worse than I do. On some days I let it bring me down so much, that staying in bed and sulking in my illness feels like the only thing I can do and really only know how to do in that moment. But you know what? I am done with using cancer as an excuse to not live. I'm not being completely insane and unrealistic though, thinking I'm not going to have those days where I just need rest would be crazy. Although I've come to these realizations, I still get that I'm sick and obviously not 100% health wise. However, I'm done blaming the cancer. I am stronger than that. I am wiser and far more determined and more fierce then this pest in my body will ever be. I choose my future. I decide how I want this journey to go. This cancer is no longer going to dictate to me in any way. It is just a road block. Uhh yeah, maybe a slightly bigger one than imagined but that's all I will ever let it be is just that, a nuisance that I will continue to face and beat down. This cancer is no match for me...I know it is going to try hard as hell to bring me down and defeat me mentally, physically and who knows how else. It has NO CLUE who it has decided to mess with. I used to be a lot weaker but my perspective has changed, as I grow in life and as a person, I will only get stronger. Until next time...

Cancer Blows, Except When It Helps

By Marilyn Geer Rivera

I knew I was sick. I could feel it the way I felt cold, the way I felt hot. I don't know how, but I knew I was dying. It was bad when I started to doubt myself, when I was told to seek mental help. I thought I had hit rock bottom, I had made a bad call, was dealing with the repercussions, fighting them actually, and I was ordered to go see this doctor one day, one that I didn't want to go see. She started asking me about my past visits and unresolved symptoms, and I just wanted to run away and actually act crazy.

When the ultrasound technician tried too hard to keep her face from showing emotion, I knew. When I had my biopsy and saw the large bruise, I knew it was cancer. When I heard it was Medullary, I had a flashback to nursing school and my instructor telling us about the different thyroid cancers, and how we would never see Medullary or Anaplastic ever, because they were so rare. I know what rare means. No money, no research, no cure.

I have always been behind the curve ball in life, I didn't have the best start, but I would be a fool to blame all my bad choices on that. I have always felt behind, even though I rushed through life. I am complicated that way. Cancer didn't focus my life at first; it just made me mad, like seriously have I not been through enough? I was going to rebuild myself, until I found another lump and I was like, "Who am I kidding, this me is the best thing I got going". I have always known what I wanted to do with my life; I just didn't have the courage. Ironically before this I had the courage to raise my right hand, to be ready to deploy to face our nations enemies, but not courage to face my secret goals. That's changed knowing for real this will kill me some day, now I feel like I am in a race against time, to check off these goals, to live my story, to add as many pages as I can to it, to be more than my cancer, to be me.

Find Joy In The Journey

By Carolyn Willis

It was 1995. I was 53 years old. My husband and I and my sister's family, my brother's family, and our dad, age 82, went on a guided trip on a motorized raft trip down the Colorado River. Between us we had six children with us, all in their 20s. It was truly an unforgettable experience, and we had so much fun! The six cousins have always had a special bond, thanks to my mom and dad, who made it their mission to bring the family together as often as possible in spite of living miles apart.

Fast-forward 20 years to New Year's Eve 2014 in Sun Valley, Idaho. With the exception of my dad (he and my mom passed away within months of each other at age 95), the same family group was together again. Over the years we had added six spouses and 14 children (including my four grandchildren). After a day of skiing we spent New Year's Eve together playing games, dancing and laughing.

So, you may ask, what does this have to do with Medullary Thyroid Cancer?

Answer: I've had sporadic MTC since 1995. I am not and never will be cancer free. My calcitonin is steadily rising. But I have been very, very fortunate to have *felt* cancer free for the past twenty years. My message, especially for the newly diagnosed, is that it's possible to live a happy, normal life with this disease. Keep your loved ones close and do your best to find joy in the journey.

A Wild Ride

By Anita Wright

My husband and I were preparing to celebrate our 43rd wedding anniversary in 2004. The day before we were leaving, I was to receive my thyroid biopsy report. I had had all the tests and scans the year before, and there had been no problems, so I was not concerned. Although I felt like something had grown (my nodule), it still was not a concern. I was retiring at the end of the school year and everything was falling into place.

WHAM! My biopsy showed papillary cancer. I was told that this was very simple to eliminate, with surgery set for the Friday before Labor Day. I would be out three weeks and should not have any complications. The hardest part was telling our children, who lived ten hours away. They were very supportive and had questions for the doctor, who was accessible and answered all.

Before surgery I was very open with the faculty, family, and friends. I worked the day before surgery. My class was stunned that I would be gone for three weeks, but they survived.

My surgery went well and they were able to remove my whole thyroid. Afterwards, I could talk, but felt woozy. The next morning I still didn't feel great. After another IV, which I failed to question, I went home with strict instructions about numbness around my mouth.

Sunday was a normal day, but Monday I woke to that dreaded numbness around my mouth. A call to the doctor and a trip to the emergency room found me back in the hospital with calcium deficiency. Two days later I was home again with my body producing calcium. I progressed quickly, although my voice was very weak and I had no pitch. I returned to teaching, using a mic and amplifier. I ordered a Chatter Vox, and this was definitely an asset.

The trip back to the doctor for my follow-up was a shock. My biopsy was wrong, as I really had medullary thyroid cancer (MTC). A calcitonin test showed it was 700. A CT-scan showed no tumors, but it did show an adrenal adenoma. A reference to another doctor an hour and a half away was made, and he ordered more tests. My calcitonin was up to 1,000 and all my other tests were normal. I was told I was sporadic and my options were to have a neck dissection or a second opinion. I was not opposed to surgery, but the doctor wanted me to have a second opinion.

Off to another surgeon, three hours away. He ran his own tests, where my calcitonin was now 1,092. He scheduled a liver biopsy, which was positive in one node.

I had several PET scans, MRIs, and CT-scans, but no tumors showed on any of these. Because of changes in the way the calcitonin was read, my numbers were now close to 600. My CEA had gone up from 84 to 92. I felt very fortunate that this was not high and I have been able to live a normal life.

After retiring, I continued to travel to my doctor every six months, because my numbers were fluctuating up and down between 100 and 200. I was now only returning to the doctor every two years, and was having him monitor my numbers from a lab closer to my home.

Another whammy hit me two months after my last scans took place. I had breast cancer. After much deliberation and family support, I chose to have a mastectomy due to an aunt who had had breast cancer. No treatments were needed, as the cancer was contained. I am carefully monitored every year with a mammogram and visit to my breast surgeon.

Things moved along with my returning every two years until I learned my doctor was moving to another hospital too far away for me to travel at this time. My personal physician is helping me monitor my numbers.

I will find an MTC specialist if my numbers double, but until then I stay active with senior aerobics three times a week and a social exercise class on Tuesday and Thursday. I am also an active member in a Canasta group, which provides my laughing therapy, and a quilting group. I sing in the choir and help with Wednesday night meals at our church. A supportive family, especially my husband, relatives and friends help me to stay in perspective. I even have a support group which I update with each doctor visit. This proves to be very important in follow-up visits. Reading their encouraging notes has helped tremendously.

Although I begin to think about my numbers several months before my twice-a-year blood work, I try to stay busy and keep my mind occupied with other things. Laughter plays a big part in my outlook. I try not to stress out, but have had several stressful times with the sudden accidental death of a grandson and my husband's two surgeries.

Since I was diagnosed, several drugs have shown success in treating MTC. There is hope! People have lived for forty years. In forty years I will be over 100!

Stand Up Straight And Keep Smiling

Anonymous

I'm a retired M.D., and as a sophomore medical student, my classmates and I developed "sophomore medical student syndrome." It's during the second year Pathology course, when medical students start learning about disease processes, including symptoms, their usual course, physical findings, laboratory findings, and so forth. Second year medical students often think they recognize all these symptoms in themselves and they fear they're developing whatever they just read about, such as brain tumor, hepatitis, or heart disease. This is the "sophomore medical student syndrome." In time, helped by denial, we moved on. As we witnessed serious and tragic illness in others, we unconsciously denied the realization that we, too, could get sick. Sickness might happen to others, but not to doctors.

Denial helps us through the tough times.

As I became elderly, I realized that something serious was waiting for me, and I again developed the sophomore medical student syndrome. Every little ache or pain made me wonder if it was the start of something big. I told myself I wasn't afraid of death, but I didn't want to look stupid, didn't want to miss my own diagnosis. I remained totally healthy. My blood pressure was 130/70. My cholesterol was under 150, my EKGs and Chest X-rays were negative. I saw my doctor once a year, with nothing to report.

My denial was working great!

A few days after my 75th birthday I found a lump in my neck. I looked in the mirror and noticed that this lump would jump up from behind my sternum (breast bone) when I swallowed. I knew it was a thyroid nodule. My primary care doctor saw me that day and wasn't impressed, but sent me to a head and neck surgeon (ENT) the next day. The ENT shooed me across the hall to an endocrinologist, who did an ultrasound and a fine needle aspiration biopsy (FNA). The biopsy was indeterminate. My ENT drew a calcitonin on the off chance that this nodule was Medullary Thyroid Cancer (MTC). My calcitonin level was 5,290. Yep, I had MTC for sure.

I was shocked. My life had changed in two weeks! After 75 successful years, denial had failed. I underwent total thyroidectomy, bilateral central compartment neck dissection, and left lateral selective neck dissection. After the operation I couldn't swallow and needed a feeding tube. Another blow to my magical thinking.

My ability to swallow returned in about three months, and my disease has been stable for almost three years. Cancer has taught me to enjoy each day as a gift. I'm very grateful for this insight, oddly grateful for the cancer. Right now my journey is easy, as I feel well and have no pain. I have resolved to stand up straight and keep smiling, no matter what.

Here's hoping!

Sonia And Marc

By Sonia Prud'homme

Aujourd'hui, j'ai tout simplement envie de dire à mon homme combien je l'aime et le remercier d'être là pour moi...'In good times and bad times', avec Marc Gaudet.

Today, I simply want to say to my man how much I love him and thank him for being here for me. 'In good times and bad times', with Marc Gaudet.

We're Not Done Yet!

By Virginia Skilton

Being the only girl with four brothers should have prepared me for all that life would have dealt out, but at age 62 I was going to find out what life had in store for me in a *big* way.

After thyroid surgery I was told I had medullary thyroid cancer (MTC). That's all I was told, other than that it was a terrible cancer. I might need more surgery and I would probably need a tracheotomy, a feeding tube, and may experience serious destruction to my neck and upper chest. I found out from the hospital and laboratory reports that I had a Stage 3 cancer diagnosis.

Stage 3? That sounded like a death sentence. Stage 4 was death, wasn't it? There was no explanation from the doctor about my staging, and his not explaining it to me at that appointment left me baffled to this day. Why?

My husband and I were in shock and left the office in tears. We started our drive toward home. Part way there I said we should go tell our oldest son what we'd been told. We were quite stoic when we broke the news to him about my cancer and prognosis. It hadn't even begun to sink in for me, let alone for my husband and my son. We left his house and drove to our other son's home. We told him in much the same way, trying to stay positive and not show how we were really feeling.

Then we headed home. At this point, what do you say to your spouse of 42 years? Do I go through with this whole process? Will I need another surgery? Do I go to a large teaching hospital like my local general surgeon recommended because he really didn't know much about my kind of cancer? He'd only heard of it, and the local hospital had never even had a case diagnosed there. That was so scary for me to contemplate. How do I do this? I didn't think of myself as a strong person because I'd always had my husband as my rock. How do I do this and possibly end up dying? What would he do?

So many questions, and hardly any answers. My head was spinning and my heart was hurting. That night I don't even remember having dinner, but I do remember when we went to bed. We held each other in our arms and cried. Cried for the future and what I would probably miss, how we would miss each other. There were so many thoughts running round and round. I don't remember if we slept much that night, or some of the nights after that. Fear of the unknown is very powerful, believe me. I was trying to rely on my faith at this point, and digging deeply for it.

Telling our family and friends was very difficult. It was like stabbing a knife into an open wound, but I tried to stay upbeat while all the time I was hurting so badly and thinking of all that I would miss if this cancer took me too soon. I loved all these people so very much and I could see by their reactions that they were hurting, too.

After many doctor appointments and tests I was scheduled for further surgery on my neck. A modified radical (that word is terrifying) left neck dissection. I'd never been a vain person, but this idea of having my neck "dissected" (sounded like a lab experiment in high school) made me wonder what I would look like. Lots of thoughts were running around in my head. Who to talk to? Who could help? I found out that at that time there was no one I knew who had this disease. I worried about what I would do if my scar was so bad it would gross people out, or scare my grandchildren. So many people knew someone who had had their tonsils or gall bladder or appendix removed, but I didn't know one person with MTC. I was trying so hard to lean on my faith, but it was hard to face my own possible demise.

So very hard. Would I be up for this? Would I be strong enough? I decided to "suck it up" and be strong.

Two months after my thyroidectomy, after I'd had some lymph nodes removed, they found there was cancer in half of them. The incision didn't look too bad, as the surgeon used glue on the outside to seal it. It extended from just under my left ear to across the middle of my neck. This was going to be a pretty sight! I had a drain at the end of the tube that went into my incision. It hung down to my breast and pulled on the incision. I thought something needed to be done about that encumbrance.

I went home the second day after surgery, with instructions on how to deal with the drain. I had to measure the liquid that drained into the bulb. Not too bad. I fixed the dangling bulb by using a safety pin and looping the hose of the drain through the pin and pinning it up on my shirt. That helped. I told myself to keep that in mind for the next time. (I hoped there wouldn't be a next time!) My chest hurt, as if the whole surgical team had stood on it during surgery. My back also hurt. I think they must have had my head hanging off the surgical table. Ouch!

Since I had MTC that meant there had to be genetic testing to see if I had sporadic or genetic medullary. This required a visit to the genetic laboratory attached to the large, well-renowned hospital where I'd had the second surgery. I really like my surgeon. He was very thorough and gentle. Nice traits for a surgeon to have.

We had an appointment with the genetic counselor and genetic doctor. When we got to the building there was a strict privacy policy. We had to wait in the lobby downstairs and were called on a phone to a certain extension and then had to wait for someone to come and escort us to the office. It seemed over the top for security, but I guess genetics is a very specific research area, and we were on their turf, and they didn't want anyone to compromise their research with our DNA.

I liked our counselor immediately. She was kind and knowledgeable about medullary and what genetic marker testing would be done for us, and that if I had the genetic mutation, then my family needed to all be tested. She collected all the medical information I could share with her about my grandparents, both maternal and paternal, my parents, my three surviving brothers, and the son of my deceased brother. I told her everything I knew and felt I had a good amount of information, since my extensive family all lived fairly close and we are all involved in each others' health histories. With the DNA testing and all the information from me she was going to put together a catalog that would tell me where they thought a defective gene had come from. At that time I was also dealing with the health insurance and getting approval for this DNA testing and further counseling appointments. This genetic possibility could have a huge impact on my family. I counted more than 70 people who might have to be tested, and then have surgeries if they tested positive for the gene. Wow, what an emotional burden!

So now all we needed to do was wait. And wait. And wait.

Almost five weeks later our counselor called me to come back for an appointment. I was informed I had the genetic marker, and what that meant.

Oh man, I hated this news! By this time I'd been doing some reading, so I knew a little about what this diagnosis could mean for my family. The next step was to have my children, brothers and nephew tested. Then we would wait again. And again. And again.

It took about a month for the results to come through. It was a good news/bad news day. My three children had each inherited the genetic marker. My brothers and nephew were all negative, so that—along with the rest of the family never having had a thyroid cancer diagnosis—meant that I was the *de novo* case. I was the only offspring from my parents to have the gene. Can I say how much I hate that I'd passed it onto my children?

Let me tell you how much I wanted these children. My whole life all I ever wanted to do was be a mother. I played with dolls until my last doll the Christmas I turned 13. I still have that doll. I used to play with my dolls in our front yard. My friend and I would haul all the doll things out to a blanket and sit under the huge maple trees in the shade and spend the day role-playing with our dolls. This set the stage for what I wanted for my future.

Something prophetic later came to light, in that my future husband was in a car with his older brother, driving down the road I lived on to see a neighbor girl whom his brother was dating. My husband remembered seeing me out there in the yard with my dolls. Another thing we put together later was that my father, who was a carpenter, had at one time remodeled my future in-law's kitchen. He remembered seeing this young boy there. Little did he know that that boy would be his future son-in-law.

Fast forward about eight years and my friends and their boyfriends decided I needed to be fixed up with someone on a blind date. The guys were both working together at this point, and my blind date worked with them. All three couples went on this date, and the rest is history.

My husband and I had both always wanted children. We shared a dream for a family. During the first two years of marriage we both had multiple tests for fertility. My husband actually had a surgery to help us get pregnant. Nothing worked, so the doctors told us they couldn't do anything more. Many tears were shed over the disappointments of testing, trying to conceive, and then the dreaded monthly period would show up. So we decided to adopt. After doing lots of paperwork, getting interviewed and collecting reference letters, we were ready for the meeting of the families who wanted to adopt. While waiting for the next and final step of interviewing, I missed my period. We were so happy! Now, to hold onto this pregnancy for the full term.

We went on to having three children of our own in two and a half years! I had three children under two and a half. Wow! I got to be a mom in a big way, in a short amount of time. They were my life. They were all I'd ever wanted and dreamed of.

The diagnosis of MEN2a with MTC was devastating, to say the least. Now that my three children had the gene they needed to have the thyroid surgery. The summer following my diagnosis my sons, who lived close by, were both scheduled the same day for their surgery. The results were that they both had MTC. One son also had papillary thyroid cancer. I sat and shook my head. I could hardly believe it.

We knew that my youngest son's two children were also positive. Our daughter, who lived out of state, had been tested and she was also positive. Her three children were tested, and two were positive. Our eldest son's boys were tested and were thankfully negative. Later the same month we traveled out of state for my daughter's surgery. It was successful and several days later her surgeon called with her pathology. She had cancer, too! Three of our precious children had this genetic marker, and now they all had MTC. Our youngest son also had papillary, and would have to do the RAI treatment.

We stayed with our daughter for almost a week. I hated to have to come back home, as I knew she could have used our help for a longer time. We planned to return the next month because both her children were scheduled for their thyroidectomies.

A month later we were back. It was a tough day for my daughter, as her children, aged eleven and nine, both underwent surgery, one after the other. It made for a very long day of worrying. They did well and there was no sign of cancer. Our grandson had some calcium issues for a couple of days, and then was sent home. No cancer was found. Finally, something to celebrate!

They were so young to have to have this surgery and then a lifetime of further testing, daily medications and the possibility of other health issues from adrenal tumors, which were a possibility with this genetic marker. My heart hurt this whole year. It was like someone sitting on my chest. Must be grief. That would make sense, wouldn't it?

There was a span of time before we had to be in a hospital again for one of the last of the two kids to have total thyroidectomies. Our nine-year-old granddaughter was the next candidate for surgery. She did well and recovered quickly. The other kids at school were curious about her scar, and she was so awesome about telling them about it. We were so proud of her. When her pathology report came in we learned that she had what was called micro-medullary thyroid cancer. They were hoping they got it early enough. She would need to be checked regularly by the pediatric endocrinologist at the large teaching hospital where the rest of us from Ohio had been treated. This diagnosis for her was so heartbreaking, as one of our precious grandchildren had cancer. I didn't care if it was "micro." It was still cancer. Would she be okay? How would our grandchildren deal with having their own children? What would be the technology to help them so that they wouldn't have to pass on this gene to their children?

I think about this so much. More heartache. Trying to hold it all in and put a positive face out there for everyone else, but my nights are troubled.

The parents of the last grandchild to have the gene wanted to put off the surgery for him as long as they could. He was only six years old, but it was his sister who'd just had her surgery and had the micro-medullary. I thought it was enough of a worry that they decided to go ahead with the surgery even though they wanted to wait. I tried hard to keep my opinion to myself, but I secretly hoped that they would decide soon.

The surgery was scheduled for our little guy during Christmas break. We were all at the hospital and waited the long hours for the surgery to be finished. He did well and didn't complain much. What troopers he and his sister had been! None of the grandchildren cried or fussed when they had to have blood drawn. I was so proud of them.

The last of the thyroidectomies was done for everyone. Out of the eight of us with the genetic marker, six of us had cancer. Two of us had papillary along with the medullary. Three had medullary with normal calcitonin. One had to do the RAI treatment one time. We all are now stable at almost five years from diagnosis. Our family has learned that we can get through the worst challenges together. We've kept the faith at whatever level we had. Prayers were asked and answered. Strength was gained from this experience, and we knew we loved each other and that love could get us through the worst days.

We keep up with our regular medical testing and follow-ups, and know this is what we must do. We thank God that we're all here today and we can lead active lives.

I know there's nothing more precious to me than my children, grandchildren and the man who made it all possible for me, my husband. The man who went on a blind date with me when he was 20 years old and I was 16. We have been a couple for 51 years, and have been married for more than 48. We've been through the worst and we have the best, and we feel blessed with a wonderful family. Our goal from the start was and always will be our precious family till we're done.

And we're not done yet!

Six Postings

By Rob Bohning

- Bill and Ashley:

I love what both of you said! Awesome reminder that there are no losers with this disease. When it's my turn one day…Nobody will tell me I lost. I give this disease the finger every day when I get on my bike and ride. And I love that your dad took cancer down with him, Ashley. It's perfect. Bill and Ashley, God Bless. We all press ahead as fighters and are not going down easily.

Rob

- Photography and the Bigger 'Picture' of Life.

I am not really much of a writer, as I usually let my photography speak for me. But as the year has progressed along, there are some things that cannot be expressed merely through photos and images, so on this New Year's Eve I will share these with you. First of all, for those of you who have been following my photography site throughout 2011, this is also a chance to meet you and introduce myself. I want to thank you all for taking this journey of photography with me, as it is not something to keep to oneself, but instead it is meant to be shared!

2011 has been a year like no other, both behind the camera, and also away from it. My Dad, who was a huge fan of my photography, battled bladder cancer since 2010 and continued this year. He passed away on September 2. Before I could catch my breath and grieve that loss, I was faced with another setback and shock. I found out the night before, on Sep 1, that I also have cancer. My first thought was, "Is this really happening?" I was adopted by him at a very young age, and there is no trace of cancer in either bloodline. But I had to accept the diagnosis that the doctors told me which is a stage IV Medullary Thyroid Cancer, a very rare and tricky cancer. This all was the result of a small bump on my neck that I asked my doctor about, and I never felt sick, not even for one day. This kind of news shifts your priorities and thoughts in a hurry.

I had an 11-hour surgery in September and the entire thyroid and 50 lymph nodes in the neck have been removed. I am very thankful to have expert doctors at the University of Texas, MD Anderson Cancer Center, who have treated many from all over the globe with this disease. In March or April of 2012 I am set to have another complete neck surgery to remove more affected lymph nodes, as multiple surgeries is the only true "cure" for this cancer. So I have re-developed my "warrior" attitude that I had during my days in the USMC. I will need it to fight this.

I write this today to encourage you all to enjoy each day under the sun and to enjoy life. Do not sweat the small stuff (and there is LOTS of small stuff)! Take things one day at a time. Trust God, love your family and spend LOTS of time with them, tell your loved ones OFTEN that you love them, and treat others with respect and love. When unexpected things happen…BREATHE!! Remember to make memories and TAKE YOUR CAMERA everywhere you go. Some of the best images I have taken are from where opportunity and preparedness have met. So don't leave it at home. Thanks for coming on this journey with me, and I plan on sharing many more images with you throughout 2012 and beyond. Happy New Year, and God Bless.

"Be still, and know that I am God." - Psalm 46:10

Rob

- Transparent Moment

I would be lying if I said I have not considered tapping out over the past several months. But will I? Not only no, but hell no. But in having two liver operations, sandwiched in the middle with a complete bilateral adrenalectomy, radiation to the liver, CT scans, MRIs, endoscopy, and colonoscopy, and more MDA famous blood sticks, the thought was tempting at times. Mostly because I have gone from 200 lbs down to 160 since January. All the brawn is well, gone. Thanks to Cushing's. For the past several months I have had indescribable fatigue and periods of abdominal pain that last anywhere from minutes to 8-9 hours. Never thought at 45 years old that my most important daily aspirations would be to get out of bed and strive to eat a 2000-calorie diet. Yes, some days I was lucky to consume 300 calories. My inter-abdominal tumors are causing a mechanical problem with my stomach. It can be cruel to live in the Texas Hill Country and take no part in the barbecues. But I press on. The days of sucking shit Jello and eating broth are over. Today, I had a full jalapeno cheeseburger, and a bowl of mashed potatoes on the side. Yep, I got all of it down. I am paying for it tonight some, but it was worth it. I am not bitching, please don't take it that way. Just saying it like it is. Here I am, and here is the situation at hand. So here I go, pressing on, and never saying die.

- Nothing Going On

Spent today at MDA…not sure how to compare days when there to something else…Like maybe reaching your hand into a box of candy and not sure what you're gonna get, but you know you will get something interesting. Anyways, met with the phase 1 clinical trial team, had blood work and a chest x-ray. 2 weeks ago I was hospitalized there for severe diarrhea, fatigue and nausea. They told me today that a urinalysis from that hospital stay shows I tested positive for an infection called Legionella. (Legion because they are many, no just kidding lol). But it can be serious and fatal. So I had one week of antibiotics, and today's chest x-ray shows much improvement from the one 2 weeks ago. The lung biopsy from 2 weeks ago still shows negative for fungal pneumonia, tumor, or bacterial pneumonia. So looks like inflammation in the lung. I will go back in 2 weeks for more blood work and chest CT. Will resume both chemo drugs tomorrow night. And getting ready for the Y90 liver procedure in June and July. Other than all that, there is absolutely nothing going on...

- Where Did These Thoughts Come From?
  So a few things to consider before flying for ThyCa:

  1. How to get my syringe through security (it is for an emergency situation in case of an acute adrenal crisis. I had both adrenals removed in June.

     TSA AGENT: "You can't take this on the plane, sir"

     The right answer:

     ME: Sir, here is my documentation from my doctor and a letter from the airline

     The wrong answer:

     ME: Dude, I don't need a syringe or a box cutter if I wanted to really do some damage.

  2. How to get my tincture of Opium through TSA.

     TSA AGENT: "This is a controlled substance and a heavy narcotic, you cannot carry it"

     The right answer: Sir, I take this as a prescription for massive, and sometimes uncontrollable diarrhea. Here is the prescription and doctor's letter for it, along with a letter from the airline.

     The wrong answer: Hey man, if I don't take this with me, both you and the flight attendant who clean up the mess are going to be hating life.

- Words

    Awesome=awe + some = some awe, means really great

    Awful= awe + full = full of awe, but yet means really bad

    So some awe is good but full of awe is really bad. Silly English language. I don't know why I am posting this, except that I have felt both this week, several times.

Joni's Journey

By Joni Eskenazi

Doctor, I said, there's a lump in my neck,
By the time of my visit, I was really a wreck,

"Don't be so concerned, it will soon go away,
Just a lymph node that's swollen," was all he could say,

But time does not heal all the problems we face,
My life now seemed in a worrisome place,

After testing concurred that surgery was needed,
To remove my thyroid, and be well... so I pleaded,

TT was performed, with biopsy showing,
I had MTC...without even knowing,

The date was August nineteen hundred ninety nine,
Information was scarce, as ThyCa started to shine,

Soon we determined that Seattle was lacking,
An experienced Doctor with MTC backing,

With the research and help of my three wonderful sons,
We headed to St. Louis, (Dr. Jeffrey Moley), it was quite a run!

We again made the journey, in October of that year,
Central neck dissection, liver laparoscopy, what more could I fear?

Referred to it then as a, "Dr. Moley Special", indeed,
My life back on track, it was time to proceed,

But, while healing I learned that our medical group,
And the funds that were needed, would not be recouped,

I was told I was required to stay with their staff,
Any ENT could have done this, now time for a laugh!

"Just a routine surgery like all others we do",
By now I knew better, who would, wouldn't you?

And so it began, my recovering days,
Fighting for rights, I was now in a haze,

Following hearings, mediation, and many denials,
Arbitration proved worthy of my now growing files,

With the knowledge and guidance of my attorney son,
They finally listened and our case was now won,

During this time, lots of questions and answers,
I was told by my Endo, "this was the good cancer!"

Laughable now, but as true as can be,
I was "fired" by an Endo, who denied treating me,

Following usual testing and several more scans,
In two thousand and twelve, and not in my plans,

More nodes were discovered too close to leave in,
To my jugular vein, the margins were thin,

I was okayed for referral outside of our plan
To see Dr. (Richard) Ball, a most brilliant man,

He concurred with the findings and suggested more tests,
To determine that surgery, might likely be best,

An FNA was instructed and performed in my group,
Once again Dr. Moley was back in the loop,

Surgery successful, once again on my way,
This time without question, my group they did pay!

Fast forward to now and new ultra sound testing,
Show nodes on the right side, my neck is not resting,

Now once again, watching and waiting to see,
While hoping and praying those nodes will leave me,

In so many ways, I feel fortunate and blessed,
To have watched the new findings, considered the best,

And watching in awe as our ThyCa does grow,
We're moving in directions that help us all know,

We are together as one, not alone anymore,
Research is helping to get to the core,

One day in the future we may hopefully see,
A cure for thyroid cancer, please join in with me,

Hang in there with hugs and hope in our heart,
As together we move, no longer apart,

Sending love to the many wonderful friends that I've made,
Very special indeed, and ones not to trade.

I look forward to meeting many more of you soon,
At the Conference in St. Louis, I'll be over the moon!

Five Generations

By Teresa Fountain

I was born in 1965 in Indiana in a middle class home life, great parents & 2 brothers, one younger brother & one older, so, yes, I was the middle child, and the only girl.

We were all healthy, besides the normal childhood illnesses.

Time passed, my brothers & I became adults, I got married & had my first child, a son, & life was humming along.

In the Spring of 1985, my mother received a letter from the Wisconsin State Board of Health stating that her birth mother located in Eau Claire, Wisconsin had a serious life threatening illness and this letter stated that my mother needed to see her Dr. immediately for a screening for a strange illness called, Multiple Endocrine Neoplasia 2A which causes Medullary Thyroid Cancer.

Yes, my mother was adopted at young age, & soon after her adoption, she moved to Indiana & my Mother never knew her birth parents, so, getting this strange letter was upsetting to my Mother, so, she threw the letter in the trash, but, thankfully, my Father rescued the letter.

Within about 10 days my mother had an appointment to see Drs. & CT scans of my mother's neck were done, & back in 1985, there were no other tests for screening the strange disease, & the Drs. were researching while my mother's CT was being processed.

Well, in a few days, my mother's surgeon had CT results, & it showed thyroid nodules, & he scheduled a thyroidectomy & the pathologist was going to do a frozen section on the thyroid tissue once the thyroid was removed to confirm if my mother indeed did have this odd cancer & weird disease called Multiple Endocrine Neoplasia 2A Syndrome.

Surgery Day arrived, my mother went into surgery & our entire family gathered in the waiting room and after an hour, about midway into the thyroid removal, the surgeon came out to let us know that he had removed the right thyroid lobe first & that my mother indeed had Medullary Thyroid Cancer & that he needed to proceed to remove the entire thyroid because Medullary Thyroid Cancer invades the entire thyroid gland system & it's an aggressive thyroid cancer with no cure, except surgery.

Once my mother's surgery was completed, and in the recovering process, we announced to my mother, that she did indeed have thyroid cancer, & the surgeon, Dr. Tierney, advised my brothers & I that the 3 of us siblings needed a special medical test done, called, "Pentagastrin Stimulation" (remember this is 1985) this was the ONLY lab test at that time to identify Medullary Thyroid Cancer.

We were all just stunned, with no symptoms, no signs or warnings, we were stunned as a family that all of this was happening. None of us were sick, but, so thankful that she had been notified by Wisconsin State Health Board that her birth mother had this strange illness.

A few months passed, and my mother recovered from her thyroid surgery and my father & she had planned a trip to go up north to Wisconsin to meet her birth mother. They went and had a great visit & my mother met brothers and sisters she never knew of, and found out that her birth mother as well as a brother in Wisconsin also had had their thyroids removed because of this Medullary Thyroid Cancer.

Soon after my parents returned from their Wisconsin visit, it was time for my 2 brothers and I to take these odd named tests called "Pentagastrin". So, I went first, & the pathologist, the lab techs, and Drs. performed this Pentagastrin in a special observation room in day surgery because these tests had never been done before in the Indiana hospitals where we lived. I clearly remember that day, I had an IV line placed in each arm, with IV fluid drips going very slowly, and the medical staff, pathology, and Drs. reading the directions out of a medical manual as they began this Pentagastrin Stimulation Test. I was not one bit nervous or afraid, after all, I stepped up to go first, my two brothers wouldn't step up, so I did.

As the testing began, the Medical staff injected a syringe of some form of IV push calcium into the right arm IV site and timed it into three to four intervals and the same drawing blood out of the left arm IV site at timed intervals, which this was a way to identify if Medullary Thyroid Cancer was present. I remember how uncomfortable that test was. It made me flush, & made my heart race; it was a terrible feeling, but, it didn't last long. Remember, this is still 1985.

My brothers and I completed these Pentagastrin tests, and within a week the surgeon called my brothers and I into his office to announce that two of us had to have thyroidectomies because the Pentagastrin tests came through as my older brother and myself appeared to have high levels of this hormone called "calcitonin" which meant we did have Medullary Thyroid Cancer. So, our surgeries were being scheduled, but, thankfully, our little brother was negative and didn't need surgery.

So, it was time and my surgery date arrived. It was September of 1985, and I was set to go and have my surgery, and there it was, I had a thyroid full of cancer, just as my mother had just a few months prior. My older brother had his thyroid removed so did I and we recovered well and we were told that we were very fortunate and that we were cured, but, also needed to be monitored and that we were to take thyroid medication every day for life! So, that was simple I thought, and I felt so thankful that we were all found and notified by the Wisconsin State Health Board.

On with life and things went well, and I finally was able to meet my grandmother in Wisconsin a few years later. It turned out that my grandmother's thyroid cancer had spread to her lungs and brain, so, I did get to travel to Wisconsin to meet her once before she passed away.

As several more years passed by, in about 1993 I found a small pea sized nodule on my right lower neck area, so I did notify my surgeon, and he blew it off and he told me not to worry, so, I didn't push it and I let it go. All I knew was that I was told in 1985 when my thyroid was removed is that I was cured.

Then a year later in 1994, the pea sized neck nodule was still there, and I was a surgical assistant in the operating room and I knew something wasn't right, so, I had asked one of the other surgeons I worked with for medical advice and he had me come to his office a few days later, and he ran blood tests called "calcitonin" and he ordered a neck CT scan.

Here I go again, my blood test of calcitonin came back very high, which meant the Medullary Thyroid Cancer was active, new recurrence, spreading, and my CT scan revealed multiple enlarged lymph nodes all over my neck, so, I was set up for surgery within 2 weeks to have an extensive neck surgery to re-open my entire neck with a procedure called a bilateral neck dissection.

I was totally beside myself, here I was 29 years old now, and I had a husband, and two children, a wonderful career in the operating room as a surgical assistant. I was devastated.

Once again, back into surgery 9 years later for neck surgery number two, it was a 5 hour surgery, with 52 lymph nodes removed and every muscle in my neck stripped down and I ended up having complications post op and ended up in ICU and such a painful recovery with 60 skin staples around my neck and 2 large drains, physical therapy, and it left me with a weak left arm due to a little nerve damage, nothing serious, but, just a little weak, but, I recovered and then I went back with living. And my post op blood tests for the calcitonin began dropping to lower numbers, which was good news.

After a few months passed by, my entire family was selected to go in with about 10 other families in the world to take part in some DNA study to see if a genetic link could be found and identified with this wacky illness called Multiple Endocrine Neoplasia which causes Medullary Thyroid Cancer and other endocrine tumors.

So, I agreed with Mayo Clinic to go in on this world study of 10 families, I wasn't sure what it was all about, but, I knew it was research and a DNA test, so, I had to practically beg my family to go in on it, so we did it and thankfully....

After about 6 months we got word from this study of the DNA, that a genetic link was identified and my family was part of a medical breakthrough, but at the same time, sadly, my twelve year old son was found to have this gene that causes Medullary Thyroid Cancer and that meant another family member was going to need a total thyroidectomy, and we were told to not wait too long to schedule my 12 year old son's surgery.

And here we go again, a 4th generation and another thyroid surgery, but, my son did very well. He had pre-cancerous Medullary Thyroid Cancer cells throughout his thyroid gland, but, caught in an early stage. So, this New DNA experiment worked out quite well. After all, it was the middle 1990's now.

Life flew by for another few years, and I began having stomach pain and nausea and high blood pressure and ended up hospitalized and once again, my calcitonin began increasing, which by now, I knew to be cancer, was making its way through my body some place again. Or did it really ever go away?

It's November of 1998 now, and, after more tests, I was sent to St Louis, Missouri from Indiana to a specialty Dr. and a team that took special interest in Medullary Thyroid Cancer. The surgeon reviewed my medical history and, he decided I needed an exploratory surgery of my abdomen, with my elevated calcitonin, which is a tumor marker for MTC. The numbers had been elevating, and my symptoms had me set up for an abdominal surgery, which meant that I would be going home to Indiana and then return and travel back to St. Louis for the surgery date.

Now, here it is December of 1998 and traveling back to St. Louis for this exploratory abdominal surgery. All kinds of emotions stirring and wondering when will this disease ever stop? And what will this surgeon in St. Louis find, and why can't my Indiana Drs. figure this out? Why did Mayo Clinic in Minnesota just blow me off and I was now ending up in St. Louis for a surgery? So, I was admitted into surgery, and had various pre op testing and then off to the operating room in St. Louis in a hospital far from home, and I didn't know anyone & in such a strange place. I had my surgery, the surgeon, Dr. Moley, found some nodules on my liver and then removed the nodules and the pathology report once again was positive for Medullary Thyroid Cancer recurrence to my liver. Now what?

This was 1998 and there was NO treatment or radiation, no chemo, nothing but just surgeries to track down and hunt down to only be removed by surgery. Dr. Moley basically explained to me and my family that this was grim news, but, I could live a year or two, or, even 10 more years? So, I swallowed that one with a gulp....

I know this illness is rare, genetic, and it's progressing and, no one seems to know what to do, so, that's when I decided to really read up and research everything I could so that I know what's going on and to get more wisdom on this rare genetic disease, because it's invading my entire family, my grandmother that I only met once had passed away & so far 4 generations of my family have this illness now. I had to be a voice and the strong one in my family and continue to do all I could do.

I recovered from my exploratory surgery and was told not much else could be done, which was okay. I was learning to live with this disease; I was drawing closer to God more each day.

Time rolled and it was the year 2001, and 2002 my son got married, & had children, so now, I got to become a grandma, and it was such a blessing.

But, I knew that my 2 granddaughters were at high risks of having Multiple Endocrine Neoplasia 2A and Medullary Thyroid Cancer. So, I began preparing and got back into my warrior research mode and began reading up on case studies around the globe with Medullary Thyroid Cancer.

I continued having abdominal pains, nausea, and was admitted to my local hospitals in Indiana and sent a few times to Indianapolis to Indiana University Medical Center's inpatient care and had a pancreas surgery, in and out of the hospitals, soon everything leveled off awhile for me, but, I was still in the research mode and I came across research documents on the internet webpage of a medical system in Switzerland that claimed to have any child tested for DNA if there are family history of Multiple Endocrine Neoplasia 2A Syndromes or for Medullary Thyroid Cancer. I read up because now I had 2 beautiful toddler granddaughters to protect.

Here it was now the year 2002, and I was hoping to God that they would not have this disease, with everything I had gone through, and I didn't want my dear granddaughters to go through all the things I had been suffering with, so we as a family decided to do the DNA testing on my granddaughters at about age one & before the girls turned 2.

Research I had found on Medullary Thyroid Cancer from Switzerland, was alarming, as it stated that many children under age five have been known to have liver metastasis, so, we as a family decided to get the granddaughters DNA, & along with a DNA, I requested the Pediatric Endocrinologist to draw calcitonin levels too, but the Endocrinologist at Riley Children's Hospital rolled her eyes and stated that kids would not have a calcitonin level at age one. My reasons, as a grandmother, and as myself living with this horrific, confusing, rare disease, were to get those little toddlers thyroids removed before cancer cells would have their way in those little thyroids, even though, the girls were 1 and 2 years old, the research I read stated that children under 5 have been known to have the Medullary Thyroid Cancer already spread to their livers, so, getting these Drs. to remove their thyroid would help. It would not give that cancer a chance to begin its invasion on their tiny bodies.

Now, a fifth generation in my family has been confirmed to have Multiple Endocrine Neoplasia 2A, and if you have this positive DNA, it's 100% you will get Medullary Thyroid Cancer. So, we press on with these little toddlers having their thyroids removed in Indianapolis at Riley Children's Hospital. They did so well, and they recovered nicely and were given a small dosage of thyroid pill daily, and just little toddlers, they took their thyroid medications every morning, just chew it up and away they go off playing like nothing ever happened to them.

The weeks, days and years are passing so fast, I was to take part in a study for Medullary Thyroid Cancer patients at the NIH, but, was taken off the study vaccine because I have rheumatoid arthritis, and it's the year 2015. I have recurrence of MTC in my liver, & several small nodules, and one 2 cm tumor in my left salivary gland. The parotid gland is enlarged, my oncologist in Bradenton, Florida, sent me to Moffitt Cancer Center in Tampa a few months back to have Moffitt Cancer Center ENT surgeons look at my neck & view my CT images to set up surgery to remove this salivary gland that's so swollen on the left jaw, neck, face. So, I went for a consult in Tampa. I thought, well good, maybe I can get into surgery to remove this left recurrent neck mass, and yes, preparing for a third neck surgery.

My calcitonin & CEA blood tumor markers are terribly elevated, which means my thyroid cancer just keeps finding its way around my body tissues. This is getting frustrating, but it is what it is, and with Moffitt cancer center in Tampa being too afraid to take me in for surgery & the NIH taking me off the cancer vaccine clinical trial, my oncologist in Bradenton, Florida was irritated as he knows I am in need of more surgery. So, what now??

My oncologist and I decided to put me on a new, rare chemotherapy agent, Cometriq, that my oncologist found. I am only one of 6 patients in the United States on this drug. I am on 100 mg a day and it's a $10,000 per month cancer drug. I prayed it would be covered by my insurance, and thankfully, yes, it was covered.

After 5 rounds of this Cometriq chemo, the usual side effects, but, my CT scans are stable, still tumors present, the main issue is my left neck, the parotid is swelling, there are lymph nodes in my neck enlarged once again, and my liver has tumor & nodules. After praying and thinking what to do, my oncologist is sending me to MD Anderson Cancer Center to a special clinic for patients with Medullary Thyroid Cancer recurrences, so we called & emailed the clinic in Houston, Texas and they want me to come out because they said, I really need to be treated, and to have more surgery.

So, here I am, after 25 plus years of living through Medullary Thyroid Cancer and 5 generations later, it's been a long journey, and I am still on the journey. I am going to do all I can to get to be part of more medical break troughs, more clinical trials, Over the past 25 plus years, I have been part of a lot of medical break troughs, and fortunately my mother's birth family found all of us.

I have been to hospitals and clinics all around this country for clinical trials, surgeries, consultations, and treatment. I have been from Indianapolis, to Minnesota at Mayo Clinic, to St. Louis, Boston, NIH, and Tampa.

So, on I go now, waiting to get to MD Anderson Cancer Center in Houston, Texas, and await a possibly third neck surgery. And as I wait, I remain on Cometriq chemo daily & being very closely monitored by my local oncologist closely until I get to MD Anderson.

Wow, what a journey it's been about 30 years and 5 generations later, it's been such a stressful, but also blessed time for us as a family.

1. My grandmother

2. My mother / her sibling

3. Myself / my Brother

4. My Son

5. My 2 granddaughters

Have all been diagnosed over the years with the RET mutation gene for Multiple Endocrine Neoplasia 2A and Medullary Thyroid Cancer. All had thyroids removed, a few family members have passed away from this illness, and some family members have or have not had any further complications or recurrences. Myself, I have had multiple recurrences and complications and as I am stage 4 now, but currently on Cometriq chemotherapy treatment of 100 mg orally, and daily. This Cometriq is fairly new, and it's not a cure, but it is treating the Medullary Thyroid Cancer and shrinking and slowing down progression. There is no real known cure, but there are clinical trials going on and hopefully, one day a cure will be found, because Medullary Thyroid Cancer behaves differently in each individual, and Drs. are not yet sure why.

I am so very thankful that we were found that my mother was found in 1985 by Wisconsin State Health Board.

As I wrote at the beginning of my memoir here, it's a miracle that we were all found, because my mother was adopted at age 3 or 4 in Wisconsin, but within a few years after she was adopted, she and her family that adopted her had all moved to Indiana and that's where she remained, we are so fortunate, because we never had any symptoms or suspicions.

And right now, I am in the process in working on a Federal Law on adopted children being found with any birth parent having genetic cancers or life threatening genetic diseases to be located. It sure saved us because Wisconsin has this state law and had it set in place way back in 1985.

On we go, I just know one day a cure will be discovered, and I am marching on with medical science & my Lord and Savior, Jesus with my family, and all my meddies, we are going to see a cure one day, real soon.

My MTC Journey

By Lois Godby

The alarm goes off, 4:30 am and time to get up and get ready for work. Hmm… the left side of my neck looks thicker than my right. I will mention that when I go for my check-up in a few days. Sitting on the exam table talking to my GP about this thickness, I see concern on her face as she examines my neck. She looks at me and says, "You know this is not good, you must get a CAT scan immediately". I thought to myself, okay, but this will be a time waste. The appointment was made quickly and results were not good, there was a large mass in my left neck and a large mass in the cecum of my bowel. Scan results stated, "Probable Metastatic Cancer." What? I am a nurse, wife, Mother, and Nana, this cannot happen!

I talked with one of the ENT doctors that I worked with and he put me on the schedule the day before Thanksgiving 2010 to do a biopsy of the mass in my neck. Well, let's get this done as I have 20 people coming to my house for Thanksgiving dinner tomorrow. The Doctor said it doesn't look good, the tumor was black, sticky and wrapped around everything in that area. My heart sank, this is real and he is talking about me. Well, maybe he made a mistake, I thought. So home I went with my husband, the ride home was very quiet, an uncomfortable silence and state of shock. No one knew I was having surgery except my husband and children, so when do I tell my sisters and other family? Thanksgiving dinner went on as planned. I did tell my sisters and again the shocked silence and then the tears. I was very stoic and no tears fell from my eyes.

Then the task of the next step. The biopsy results were in and the diagnosis was Medullary Thyroid Cancer, rare and not curable. Shut down, please don't call me or ask me if I am okay! No, I am not okay and you can't do anything for me! Please just let me go into my cocoon as I will be dead soon. More phone calls, we have to get a colonoscopy set up for you to check the mass in your bowel, possibility it could be from the Medullary. Put on my, "everything is fine" face, and go into my work and get the colonoscopy over with. Lots of hugs well wishes and sorrowful looks. Biopsy from the bowel mass back and not cancer! Thank you, God. Now to do some research. After hours and days I decided to have a surgeon from the University of Cincinnati do my thyroidectomy and any other needed surgery.

My thoughts went wild, as a surgical nurse, I knew every possible outcome and the worst weighed heavy on my mind. My big surgery day was here and my family arrived to go with me, everyone was frightened for me. I asked my nurse daughter to stay overnight with me as I was very frightened also, but never admitted that to any off them. My daughter was uncomfortable staying as she was an "oncology nurse" and knew nothing about surgical patients. I didn't want her to take care of my physical needs, just my emotional needs, and have her close by. That hurt so much when she didn't eagerly want to stay. When I went to surgery, I didn't know if she was staying or not, but in the end she ended up staying.

So much pain when I woke up, two drains in my neck and my entire sternocleidomastoid muscle, total thyroid and 53 lymph nodes from the left and 11 from central neck removed. After 3 days I was discharged home with one drain in place. Hours turned into days of severe pain in my neck and chest, after 2 weeks it settled down to manageable pain and life went on. I then received a call to get the mass removed from bowel as it may cause a blockage soon. So one month later here I was getting ready for another big surgery, a bowel resection. Spent 3 days following the surgery and when biopsy results were back, to my shock there was cancer found in the bowel mass, a totally different type, adenocarcinoma.

After the shock settled, I realized this was good news, well as good as could be, as it was a different type of cancer that meant the Medullary had not spread! After 6 months off I returned to work, my stamina was not good, overwhelming fatigue, I can't do this, it's too much. I asked for a transfer to a nursing department making phone calls and cut down to 3 days per week. I decided to search for others with my disease and found a group on Yahoo!. What a blessing and from there a group was formed on Facebook and now we are a big family of "Meddies", I have learned so much and continue to learn from each and every one.

One year after my diagnosis, my husband lost his job, at the paper company where he had worked for 44 years. It just closed its doors. My husband was 62 and I was 60, so I was now the breadwinner and carried the insurance. I felt a lot of pressure. What if I can't work, what will we do for insurance? I tried to talk to my husband about my fears but his answer was, "I guess we will have to pay for it ourselves." I looked at the numbers and that would be $60,000 over the next few years, not possible. I was so hurt that he would let me go to work with this cancer hanging over my head, instead of finding another job. Soon after, my 4th Grandchild was born, and something was wrong. She was whisked to Children's Hospital NICU and remained there for 45 days. After many heart breaking days she was diagnosed with HIE which would result in her having Cerebral Palsy. She was not able to eat and had a gastric tube placed to feed her. We were so heartbroken for her and prayed so hard all would be okay. I realized, though, that God does have a plan; my husband's job was gone so he could be the help my daughter would need when our granddaughter, Sophia, came home. Sophia has a brother, age 4, and sister, age 2 at the time, and it was impossible for Mommy to care for them without help, as Sophia needed 24 hour care. My stamina was not good and my husband stepped up and was there every day. So life has gone on and 4 years later my tumor markers continue to rise and there are scattered nodules in my lungs and my par tracheal area. I am in a clinical trial at NIH and have great hope that the vaccine they give me will show good results at stabilizing this horrible disease. I pray every day that a miracle will come, for my granddaughter Sophia, and that a wonderful cure or prevention will come along for all of us. And yes, I am still working 3 days a week with wonderful people that are indescribably kind to me and to Sophia!

God Bless.

Today Is A Good Day For A Good Day

By Tammy Vetter

My journey began with going to the doctor about a lump on the side of my neck that really itched and had been there for about six months. He told me about the swollen lymph node he has in his neck, and that it was nothing. Then he patted me on the knee and said, "Well, we'll do an ultrasound just to make you feel better." After the ultrasound he called me and was really apologetic; he said he was setting me up with an endocrinologist.

I had a biopsy and then surgery for my "papillary" thyroid cancer. I had the radioactive iodine treatments and later had a second surgery for a couple new nodes. During the second surgery my left vocal cord became paralyzed. The surgeon made me feel like I was wasting his time. After all, I just had thyroid cancer. After my second surgery I was actually told by the nurse to see my endocrinologist in a year, and if they didn't call me with an appointment I should call them. "We don't want you to fall through the cracks," she said.

I think the hardest part about telling everyone was all the free advice I got. I know they meant well, but it made me feel like I caused this to happen to me. It was all my fault because I didn't eat the right foods or take the right supplements. But now that they told me, I was supposed to start taking all this stuff and I'd be fine. I really started to pull away from people who just wanted to tell me how to cure my cancer. And if I had a nickel for every time someone said, "Well, you look good," I'd be rich!

I decided to go to Mayo Clinic in Rochester for a second opinion. I felt a little silly that I might be overreacting and wasting their time, and considered canceling many times up until the day of the appointment. They had gotten all the pathology reports from my first two surgeries, and when I got there I had numerous appointments set up. The endocrinologist I saw was really kind and asked me a few questions, then said, "You don't have papillary thyroid cancer."

My first thought was "I've gone through two surgeries and radioactive iodine treatments and I don't even have cancer!?"

Then she dropped the bomb. "You have medullary thyroid cancer. Do you have any questions?" I had never read anything about medullary thyroid cancer except that it may be genetic and was really rare. My thoughts went immediately to my children and my new one-year-old grandson. I gave them cancer!

After the testing I found out that my cancer was sporadic. I relaxed, my children were okay. I could now concentrate on having the next surgery. I joined a support group for medullary thyroid cancer, the "Meddies" on Facebook, and was so glad. I learned so much from everyone and was able to understand more about this cancer.

Also, what a difference it was at Mayo! I felt so cared for and comfortable with my doctors. I had to have a fourth surgery on my neck later that year. I was back for the follow-up appointment and they discovered new nodes in my neck and said I needed radiation because I couldn't have surgery every six months, as my neck was getting really difficult to operate on after four surgeries. The radiation was set up for six weeks of treatments.

I was so lucky to get into the Hope Lodge at Rochester during my treatments. Everyone there was going through radiation, and special bonds were formed. It was so comfortable. We all had something in common, so understood to a point what each of us was feeling. One day towards the end of my radiation I was really down and struggling. When I was checking in a little girl in a stroller was coming out. She had no hair and was waving at the nurse and smiling. That was a turning point for me. If this precious little girl could do this smiling and happy, I could surely buck up and do this, too.

When I went back for my follow-up after radiation I asked about a lump in my skull. Another biopsy. Sure enough, it was medullary thyroid cancer, which was now in my soft tissue. I had surgery to remove that. My oncologist thought I should consider the tyrosine-kinase inhibitor (TKI) cancer drug, Caprelsa.

I had earlier met a wonderful lady at the ThyCa conference in Chicago. We were like twins with our cancer. We both had about the same calcitonin and CEA numbers, and our cancer was in the same areas. She started Cometriq and didn't have an easy time. She lost a lot of weight and really felt horrible. She has since passed away, which was so hard, because we'd gotten so close in such a short time. I really miss talking to her. One of the last emails I got from her told me to stay off TKIs as long as I could. Her last words to me were in my head, and I said no to the Caprelsa at that time.

I'm now at the point where I need to start one of the TKIs, and I'll do it with the knowledge that it's going to help me. One night, I don't know where it came from, I saw this strong message in bold letters: *YOU DON'T HAVE TO DIE*! I slept with such peace that night.

So a new journey will be starting for me, and I know it will be okay.

I have a sign on the wall by my bed that says, "Today is a Good Day for a Good Day." Every day I wake up and read that is a gift from God, and I am grateful!

Life Without Parole: A Story Of Life With MTC

By Ralph Valeri

Prior to Cancer

I'm a 59-year-old male who was diagnosed with Medullary Thyroid Cancer in May of 2009. I was married in my late twenties, had twin boys, and two years later, my little girl. My wife and I raised three children whom we couldn't be more proud of. I was a loving father, a family man. I coached my kids' soccer teams, went to all their school activities, and took them on great vacations to different parts of the country every summer. Being a handyman, I was always making improvements to our home, and my mechanical abilities must have saved us a fortune on car repair and maintenance.

My true passion in life is fishing! I've been in pursuit of the Largemouth Bass since I was twelve years old. Every summer – after my fatherly duties of course – all 47 of them, I've been on the lake. I even let my boys, in their young teens; drag me through the woods, as they wanted to learn to hunt. Something I'd never done before!

My wife and I were very different personality types. But we hardly ever fought, and provided a great environment for our children. Unfortunately, over time our differences put us in the situation of just "existing" under the same roof. I wanted love and happiness and knew something had to change. As my boys went off to college the divorce proceedings began. It didn't take much time to reach a very amicable divorce.

Cancer Treatment

My cancer journey consists of love, marriage, divorce, happiness, sorrow, pain, and the struggle to just exist. Early in 2009 I began to have a strange pain in my right hamstring that wouldn't go away. My doctor suggested an MRI. The results showed a mass in the sacral bone, better known as the tailbone. A biopsy was performed and the diagnosis was Medullary Thyroid Cancer, or MTC.

In the past six years since the diagnosis, I've been on one experimental oral chemotherapy pill, and two other similar drugs approved by the FDA to fight this cancer. I've undergone three surgeries, the first to my tailbone, the second a removal of my thyroid, and then a neck surgery to repair my C5 vertebra, which had been partially destroyed by a tumor. This cancer can spread to the bone, liver, lungs, and other organs. Mine seems to be confined to the bone. Unfortunately, I have a lot of tumorous activity in my spine. I have undergone radiation treatments on four separate occasions to kill growing tumors there.

My doctor explained that this was a slow growing cancer and we'd deal with it as needed. MTC makes up only about 4 percent of the four types of thyroid cancers. Two of the thyroid cancers make up more than 90 percent of this cancer and are treatable with regular chemotherapies. MTC does not respond to these drugs because it's a slow growing cancer and acts very differently from the others. The good part of this story is that when I was diagnosed in 2009 there were no treatments other than radiation. Since then there have been two drugs approved by the FDA to specifically fight MTC, and various drugs designed to fight other cancers have been shown to slow this disease. I'll be starting on a new oral drug soon that was just approved. These drugs are not a cure. They seem to keep existing tumors from growing larger, and help keep new tumors from forming. MTC is incurable, but survivable!

In January of 2011 my doctor suggested I should get into a clinical trial for a new drug, an oral chemotherapy pill. We'll call it Drug #1. It was. It worked well for me for about a year. Then, as luck would have it, the cancer was smart enough to become resistant to the drug. In March of 2012 I started to take another oral chemotherapy pill, Drug#2, but this one was just FDA approved. It worked well to hold the cancer in check for about twenty months. At that point, early in 2014, I was put on Drug#3. It was not specifically designed for MTC, but had good results on other cancers. I've been lucky to have many treatment options become available to me in the past six years.

Here's a brief synopsis of my fight, not with the drugs but with the cancer itself. I was diagnosed with MTC in May of 2009. My tailbone surgery followed in July, and my thyroid was removed in October of 2009. Things were quiet until October of 2010, when a pain in my shoulder led to the discovery of a tumor in my T2 vertebra. Radiation was performed and the tumor was eliminated. The vertebra had slightly collapsed and was close to my spinal column. It was added to a list of things to be monitored carefully in the future. The year of 2011 was fairly normal. In September of 2012 I developed a pain in my spine that turned out to be a tumor eating away at my T4 vertebra. I had radiation in October of 2012. It was successful and the pain went away, but the bone was slightly collapsed and close to my spinal column, so it, too, has been monitored closely.

In September 2014 I had to have surgery on my C5 vertebra, which had been eaten away by the cancer. The bone collapsed and was pressing against my spinal column, causing great pain. The surgery consisted of placing a spacer in the area that had been affected and secured to the C4 and C6 vertebra with a plate and some screws. Shortly afterward, in November of 2014, I underwent radiation to a couple of tumors in my ribs on my left side. Having been taken off the latest cancer drug back in September prior to my surgery, the cancer seemed to have run wild, like it knew there was no resistance. The rib pain stayed with me for months before finally subsiding. In February of 2015 my routine CT scans showed that my C2 vertebra had signs of a tumor starting to eat away at it. I had radiation treatments to kill the disease in this area. For some reason, after this radiation my body seemed to say "enough already," and I became sick like I'd never been sick before. I couldn't eat or sleep. It took three weeks before I felt better.

The Daily Fight

The fight has gone on for six years, from May 2009 until April 2015. The 8.5-hour surgery to remove the tumor in my tailbone was successful, but left me with nerve pain in both my feet, which causes me to take pain medication to this day. My thyroid removal was a simple surgery, but living without this organ goes way beyond simple. My neck surgery, although serious as far as the spinal cord compression issue, has left me without any long-lasting effects.

I take two different types of pain medicine for the nerve pain in my feet. Without them there I'd have constant pain. I'm not sure the effect these pain medications have on my brain as far as fatigue or "brain fog" is concerned, but they seem necessary for my overall comfort. As for the thyroid gland, the sole function of the thyroid is to make thyroid hormone. This hormone has an effect on nearly all tissues of the body, where it increases cellular activity, regulating metabolism. People without a thyroid take a daily pill, which provides a synthetic replacement of the missing hormones. It takes some time to get the dosage correct, but it seems most people still suffer from fatigue. I believe this is due to the thyroid's ability to deliver these hormones as needed in the ups and downs of daily life, while the synthetic replacement is a steady dose.

The oral chemotherapy drugs have side effects that just add to the issues already encountered from other drugs, the main one being fatigue. Some refer to it as brain fog. It makes you feel like a slug all the time. In addition, diarrhea becomes prominent. Other side effects include mouth sores, overall mouth irritation, rash, acne, and sun sensitivity. It's great to have these drugs to fight the cancer, but it's a daily struggle for you to fight the drugs! Having to fight sleeping problems, depression, appetite issues and more, requires even more drugs to be introduced into the system.

It's a daily battle. Every day I feel very lethargic and fatigued. I have to push myself to do anything worthwhile. It seems that if I have to do something, I can get it done, but otherwise, forget it. Running to the bathroom always gets me moving! And then there is the constant wondering whether the drug or the disease is causing the most problems. Is it the pain pills? The anti-depressant? The thyroid medicine? The cancer drug? Or the cancer itself?

The Personal Toll

It was in the middle of 2006 when my first divorce was started. I'm not sure when it was finalized. About a year and a half later I reconnected with my childhood sweetheart. After dating for about a year, we bought a home together in January of 2009. Yes, the same 2009 during which I was diagnosed with MTC. A year later we got married.

Things were going well, or so I thought. It was January of 2011 when I started on the clinical trial for the first cancer drug. I was tired more often, but continued to work. I made sure my personal life wasn't affected too much by my fatigue. My wife and I went on two vacations in 2011 and lived pretty much the way we always had. Then came February of 2012, and the relationship issues. She had to work on a Saturday that February. A first in the whole time I knew her. That night she picked a fight with me. I expressed my dislike for her attitude, and as she was walking away I told her it would be nice if she could care about someone other than herself. I was met with, "I can't go on like this. I thought we'd be taking hiking vacations by now and things like that." I walked away, and within a few weeks, she filed for divorce.

Didn't we love, didn't we share
Or don't you even care
I know we said that we were through
But I never knew how quickly I would go
From someone you loved
To someone you used to know

I heard this song yesterday and had never equated it to this situation until now. I used to like it, but now I'm not so sure. It does fit the situation. So much for love, happiness and any kind of support.

I spent all of 2011 (the first year on Drug#1) struggling to keep our life as normal as possible. It was very hard. When I didn't feel well or was tired, I tried to downplay it because I knew I wouldn't get any sympathy. My down time meant more free time for her to do things for herself. When you feel bad and your mental state needs some compassion and caring, having some support can be the best thing for you. During the divorce, I moved out. My mother lived alone in a condo and was glad to have me. It's been three years since the day I left.

In October of 2013, I was laid off from my job of 18 years as a computer programmer. So now I'm unemployed and living with mom. I looked for work for a few months before I decided that the cancer and drugs had made me too tired to continue. In February 2014 I went on Social Security Disability. My disability pay is a decent amount of money, but I was paying a fortune to a COBRA insurance plan through my previous employer. With medical bills on top of that, buying a home was looking a little bleak. I lost a minimal support system when my wife walked away. I lost an even better support system when I was laid off from my job. Now my support system is my children, my mom, all the people at my Oncologist's office, the radiation department, the CT and bone scan department, and all my friends at the pharmacy. I can't leave out FISHING! Someone looks down over me and makes my summer months the best for my health.

Life Without Parole

I feel very lethargic every day, but I still do everything for myself, such as grocery shopping, meals, laundry, etc. I think I must be too proud to let anybody do anything for me. My doctor is starting me on a newly approved drug that hopefully will put this disease back into hiding. The past six years have been quite the roller coaster. Some highs, and a lot of lows. But I have hope. Many new drugs have been developed, and I hope there are more to come. The longer I can hang on, the more hope there is for a cure! I've experienced too much pain and heartache from this disease. They say this makes us strong, and they're right! I dragged my lethargic butt to the lake yesterday and did some fishing. While my poor body is paying for it today, I'm strong enough to handle it.

I hate this damn cancer! It's locked inside of me with no chance of getting out. In short, it's "Life Without Parole."

You're Screwed

By Karen Tesauro

My story started in 1990 when I was 28 years old. I just didn't feel right. I couldn't say this hurt or that hurt, just that something was wrong.

I've always had a chubby neck. When I was younger, my mother would take me to the doctor to have my thyroid checked, but my levels were always normal and I was told to lose weight and it would go away.

In 1993, I couldn't take it anymore and decided I had to find out the cause of my mystery illness. During an exam, a doctor felt an enlarged thyroid and a lump and sent for radioactive iodine testing. I was diagnosed with nontoxic multi nodular goiter. I was told that nodules are very common and almost everyone has nodules, so don't worry about it. It's not cancer.

In 1994, I gave birth to my daughter, Tiffany. I struggled through the next few years feeling tired and weak all the time. By 1998, I couldn't take it anymore and went on a mission again to figure out what was wrong.

I went to doctor after doctor. I was told that it is just depression, that I'm over worked, that I had a high pressure job, that I was a single parent. All you need is Cymbalta. She made me feel like I really was crazy.

Then I went to an oncologist. He literally told me, "If something was really wrong with you as many years as you say it has, you would be dead by now. You just need a boyfriend." Really? Like having sex is really the answer to all that's ailing me?

I couldn't take the humiliation of these doctors. They made me feel like I was crazy. So I gave up. At least for a while.

By 2003, I went on my next quest. I found a new endocrinologist, and she ran all of the tests again. Lab work, Radioactive iodine, ultrasound, and even a biopsy. Labs weren't too bad. Ultrasound showed enlarged thyroid with several nodules. Radioactive iodine showed non-suspicious nodules and biopsy came back benign, calcified nodules. Again, nontoxic multi-nodular goiter. And several other doctors say basically, I'm crazy.

In 2006, I started begging my endo to have my thyroid removed. My neck was getting bigger, I was having difficulty breathing and talking. I felt like I was being strangled all of the time. She said no, they don't just remove thyroids.

In May 2007, I was 45 years old. My endo noticed that one of the nodules grew quite a bit and ordered another biopsy. Guess what! A week later I received a call from my doctor's secretary saying that I have cancer and the doctor wants to see me first thing in the morning. Can you believe the doctor had her secretary give me the news? On the phone?

That night I got on the internet and read up on the different types of thyroid cancer. In my mind I categorized papillary and follicular as "oh shit, these seem fairly treatable and most common". Then there was medullary which I called, "You're screwed". Well maybe I used a different word and anaplastic was, "you're dead".

So I went to the doctor's office the next morning basically assuming I had "oh shit" because the other types were so uncommon. Or maybe, I didn't have any of them.

I was wrong. I have, "you're screwed", aka medullary thyroid carcinoma. She said, "don't worry". You still have a 10% chance to live 5 years. This probably sounds crazy, but part of me was relieved that after all these years I wasn't crazy. At least with a diagnosis it was something I could deal with.

My surgery was scheduled within 2 weeks At Jackson Memorial in

Miami. During that time, I had all of the body scans done, looking for metastatic disease. It had spread to my liver, and bones. Calcitonin was 5260 and CEA 128.

My surgery lasted 9.5 hours. The cancer had encased my left vocal cord nerve and it had to be sacrificed. I recovered well but could barely talk, and difficulty breathing due to the vocal cord. Calcitonin dropped to 1280 and CEA to 62.

I went back to work a few weeks later, but it was so hard, especially with no voice. My company was going thru layoffs due to the economy, so I didn't tell them the extent or my prognosis for fear of losing my job.

By the beginning of 2008, the pain in my lower back was excruciating. My legs ached so badly from the mets on my lower spine and pelvis. So I went through radiation to slow the growth in those areas, and it really helped. But trying to work every day, with a smile, without a voice and just trying to say a few words was like running a marathon. And was more than I could handle.

I found out that the advanced medullary thyroid carcinoma qualifies as a disability under the Social Security guidelines, so I decided to go on disability.

In December of 2012, I turned 50 years old. I was in the 10% that lived past 5 years. I now realize those statistics are a bunch of BS. But I did throw myself one heck of a 50th birthday party!

So here we are in 2015. I am one lucky girl. My cancer has grown very slowly with calcitonin around 7000 and CEA around 300.

In many ways this cancer has been a blessing in my life. It allowed me to spend my daughter's teenage years at home with her, rather than working 60 hours a week. I always wanted to get involved with charities but never had the time to help friends or stranger, and now I do.

God is keeping me on this earth for a reason and my life has more meaning and purpose than before I heard the words that mean, "You're screwed".

Four Years And Counting

By Don Olson

My journey began February 28, 2011, at the office of my gastroenterology doctor. My Dad had died in 1958 at 39 years of age from colon cancer, so I had been having screenings for more than 20 years. I had been diagnosed with gastroesophageal reflux disease (GERD) and was taking Nexium. It was time for an appointment to renew my prescription, and during that appointment the nurse practitioner asked, "What's that on your neck?"

My response was "I shave every morning and there's nothing on my neck."

She went on to tell me that there was a lump on the left side of my thyroid and recommended I get it looked at by my primary care provider (PCP). So I made an appointment to also get a follow-up PSA test. In January of 2009 I'd been diagnosed with prostate cancer and had surgery for it in September. I'm a Viet Nam veteran, so I wanted to double check to see that *that* cancer was taken care of, and the PSA test is the way that's done. On March 2 my PCP checked my neck and sent me to have a thyroid ultrasound the following day. I was assigned an endocrinologist and got an appointment for March 16.

I had blood labs and an ultrasound-guided fine needle aspiration scheduled for the next day. Five days later Dr. Fallon called, telling me he was sorry to inform me that I had Medullary Thyroid Cancer (MTC). I looked it up on the Internet and was flabbergasted. Dr. Fallon had set up an appointment with Dr. Prior, a surgeon. He had a copy of the test results and went over them with my wife and me, but wasn't much help answering our questions. He told us Dr. Fallon had also ordered more blood labs, a 24-hour urine test, an MRI and a CT scan. I did the 24-hour collection thing the next two days, but the MRI and CT scans took several days to schedule and complete.

The next several days are still quite unclear. I remember it was upsetting that CEA range *should* be < 2.5 and mine was 117, that the Calcitonin range should be < = 10 and mine was 967. *This couldn't be good*! I might as well stop paying for those AD&D (accidental death and dismemberment) insurance policies because I won't be needing them! It seemed everyone I notified of my diagnosis had a different suggestion of where to go and who to see, because they had a family member or friend who was, "Doing just fine now."

In the midst of all this chaos I got a call from my youngest brother's wife, Judy. She told me that one of her best friends had a daughter, Nicole, who had been diagnosed with MTC last year. Judy told me she had talked with Sharon and that she wanted me to call and talk with her about it. That was truly God sent, I'm absolutely certain of that.

Sharon had been waiting for my call. What a relief it was to talk with someone who had been through what I was going through and could answer some of my questions. She also asked me some questions about things I knew nothing about. *Yet.*

Sharon told me some of Nicole's journey during the previous year and recommended I see someone in a Center of Excellence for a second opinion. Nicole had been treated at Johns Hopkins and her endocrinologist there was Dr. Douglas Ball. Sharon also shared with me that there were two online groups I should look into, one on Yahoo and the other on Facebook. I had a Yahoo account so I started there and found I truly wasn't alone. What an amazing source of information and contact with others having a very similar situation in their lives. Sharon also gave me the phone number of Johns Hopkins and the email address of Dr. Ball's office assistant. I called and asked for an appointment with Dr.

Ball, and the registration person told me the first available appointment was the second week of July. I also emailed the medical office coordinator of Dr. Ball's office to introduce myself.

I saw Dr. Fallon on March 30, 2011, and he had most of the test results back. He went over them with us and was able to explain what they were all for but that the genetic test results were not back yet. He went on to explain that MTC sometimes indicates a more complex condition that affects other parts of our endocrine system. While awaiting the genetic test results he reviewed the MRI, CT scan and urine reports to see if there were tumors in other places, because MTC is known to be a metastatic disease. All the tests and scans so far were negative, meaning no problems were detected.

On April 11, 2011, Dr. Fallon called and told me the genetic results were back and I was positive. At that time I had no idea what that really meant. Two days later I was able to get a copy of the actual Quest Diagnostics Clinical Laboratory Report. It read:

RESULT: HETEROZYGOUS POSITIVE FOR A RET MUTATION ASSOCIATED WITH MEN2 OR FMTC.

Multiple endocrine neoplasia type 2 (MEN2) is an autosomal dominant genetic disorder with a high lifetime risk of medullary thyroid cancer. It is classified into three subtypes, MEN2A, familial medullary thyroid carcinoma (FMTC), and MEN2B, based on the presence of other clinical presentations. MEN2 is caused by mutations in the RET proto-oncogene." The report continued with assay percentages of detection and even process sequence steps. The most significant statement was " Mutation identification can be used to confirm a diagnosis, screen individuals at risk for familial disease, or distinguish familial from sporadic disease.

In one fell swoop I learn not only do I have an uncommon, incurable cancer, but that there's a genetic component and my whole family may also be at risk. Now don't get me wrong here, getting this report wasn't all that upsetting to me. On the contrary, getting this report gave me a better understanding of my circumstances, and "knowledge is power." In just over three weeks I went from being almost totally unaware of MTC to being told I have it and my genetic family has a high risk of it as well. I am one of five siblings and I have two grown children, so we started out with six more people who needed to be tested.

On April 13 I called a local genetic counseling office and got an appointment. They mailed me forms to fill out about my family history. On April 15, Dr. Fallon called and told me I had an appointment with Dr. Ball at Johns Hopkins on APRIL 22 at 7:45am. That was just one week away!

That next week was spent doing all kinds of Internet browsing and informing my two brothers, two sisters, and both of my two children of the genetic connection with my cancer, which was telling them that it could be *our* cancer. We always have been a close family, so there was no big problem there. Everyone understood they were invited to the genetic counseling appointment and accurate family history was important for that to be effective.

According to GPS, the road trip to Johns Hopkins is just under five hours, so we went the day before and stayed with friends who lived just 30 minutes from the outpatient clinic. April 22 was Good Friday that year, and that was truly the most significant Good Friday of my life.

During the 7:45-8:30a.m. appointment with Dr. Ball. He called Dr. Sara Pai, a surgeon otolaryngologist, to see if she had time to see me and evaluate me for surgery.

At 9:00a.m., signed in for a full neck ultrasound.

At 10:00 a.m., met Dr. Pai and set up an appointment for after the ultrasound.

At 11:00a.m., got ultrasound.

At 12:15-1:15p.m., examined by Dr. Pai to record throat and vocal cord function.

Quick break for lunch in our van in the parking ramp.

At 1:30, went to Dr. Pai's office to pick up pre-operative evaluation letter.

At 2:00-3:00, needle biopsy of "suspicious node in level four."

By 3:30p.m., on our way back home.

I read over the pre-operative evaluation letter and noticed the following: "Mr. Olson is scheduled for an inpatient procedure (thyroidectomy/neck dissection) with Dr. Sara I. Pai on Monday, May 2, 2011." WOW! Four and a half weeks from the day of my notification of MTC to the day I have a letter from a notable surgeon at a Center of Excellence for the treatment of MTC! DOUBLE WOW!

I have just one week to meet these requirements: a history and physical exam, Labs with CBC, Chem panel, PT, Ptt, Vitamin D, and Electrolytes, Chest x-ray, and recent EKG. Johns Hopkins Pre-Operative Evaluation Form was to be completed and faxed, along with Lab results, etc., to the given number, "no later than Friday, April 29, 2011. FAILURE TO FOLLOW THESE INSTRUCTIONS WILL RESULT IN THE CANCELLATION OF YOUR SURGERY." Now consider that ride home after such a wonderfully successful day and understanding the challenge before me. There were certainly peaks and valleys.

On April 25 I took the forms to my PCP's office and found he was not in. Got an email from Dr. Ball's Medical Office Coordinator and he ordered CT of neck and chest and MRI of abdomen. The next day my local Office Coordinator of Endocrinology called and told me CT & MRI scheduled for 11:00 to 1:00. I picked up copies of the two CDs of CT and MRI and delivered them to the Office Coordinator, who would make sure they got to Dr. Ball. I got a call from my PCP's nurse telling me I had an appointment with PCP at 3:00 April 27 and an appointment with genetic counselor was 3:30. I made it to PCP appointment, had EKG, constructed history. At genetic counseling appointment, I'm told my first cousins should be informed of my mutation. I have 31 first cousins. On Thursday I picked up an extra copy of the Pre-Op report and history my PCP always makes for his patients to hand carry with them to their surgery appointment.

The next day I got a call from Dr. Pai's Office Coordinator stating she had not received the blood labs, so I gave her my PCP's office number. I got a call from PCP's nurse. ASAP blood lab appointment, the Pre-Op letter had been filed. PCP and his nurse had not seen it! Twenty-five-minute trip to PCP office, blood draw, done deal. They ran the labs PDQ and fax'ed the results to Dr. Pai's office. Just in the nick of time.

On Sunday we drove to Baltimore. On Monday we got there around 8:30am for my 10:00 show up time. Surgery began about 1:30pm, duration four hours. I went to the ICU because my heart rhythm showed a bundle branch block just as they were closing. Normal rhythm returned before I actually got to the ICU. I awoke around 4:00am and was feeling good, just like I did when the lights went out some 14 hours earlier. I could swallow, turn my neck every way, and all without what I call pain. A little discomfort, maybe, but no pain. Then I realized I was hungry. I must not have been feeling any pain because all I seemed to be aware of was that it had been more than 36 hours since I had eaten anything! When my wife and family came in I asked to have some snacks. Two packages of peanut butter crackers went down the hatch by the time breakfast got there.

One of the endocrinologists from Dr. Ball's office came to check on me and told me Dr. Pai would be the one to release me with post-op instructions. Dr. Pai had minced and auto-transplanted my left and right inferior parathyroid glands into the corresponding sternocleidomastoid muscles so blood was drawn about noon to check calcium. That was okay, so I was discharged at 2:00pm and we drove the five hours home. The next day was a very welcomed day of rest. The following day I was on my way to get serum and ionized calcium blood labs taken and Dr. Pai personally called my cell phone to see how I was doing. She called again after she got the results. I have been totally impressed by the doctors and medical staff at Johns Hopkins.

Life is all about timing. When this opportunity came to share this transformative part of my life with others, some of whom are right now going through similar things, I was awaiting the latest results of my on-going blood tests to see if my MTC was stable or progressing. For those meddies on the Facebook group who are reading this, you're familiar with the term, "on the anxiety train." Well, that train ride ended night before last when Dr. Ball called to let me know my test results were in. He left the message that he would leave the test results for me on a "My Chart" message. It stated: *The calcitonin was elevated this time at 17. For comparison it was <2 in August 2013. CEA was normal at 2.1. T4 and TSH was ok at 1.3 and 0.9. Calcium was normal at 9.3. Let's plan for a follow-up visit this summer with a repeat neck ultrasound. We can get another calcitonin and CEA about a week or two before. Please contact Nickey to arrange.*

Dr. Ball is a *super* doctor and a *super, super* person. Two years ago, after my second MTC surgery, a left neck dissection, he called on a Sunday afternoon to let me know my calcitonin was less than 2, which is considered "undetectable." That call was followed up by a letter that same day that read:

We're delighted that your calcitonin has become undetectable since your surgery with Dr. Pai April 19, 2013. I'd like to recheck calcitonin and CEA in September. While it's certainly possible the values will go up again in the future, this is nonetheless a great result.

Since that last call and letter I had another <2 calcitonin and then a 3 reading, so I had gone back to almost ignoring the reality that I would probably have Medullary Thyroid Cancer for the rest of my life.

I replied to Dr. Ball's message and requested an appointment in June. I've been having increasing trouble with swallowing and with my voice the last couple of months and can't determine if it's lymph node related or not. I'm from upstate New York and we had a rough winter and spring. My MTC journey is ongoing, four years and continuing.

How Did I Get This Cancer?

By Stanley Johnson

In 1998 I was not feeling well and had a palpable lump on the right side of my neck. My primary care physician said it was just a cyst. I requested a biopsy and was diagnosed with Medullar Thyroid Cancer (MTC). My calcitonin was at 1000. The ENT referred me to an endocrinologist in Grand Rapids, Michigan. After visiting with him, he called Ann Arbor Hospital and was told the first appointment would be three months out.

The endocrinologist said no, he needs surgery *now*. He then contacted Mayo Clinic in Rochester, MN. They said they would take me immediately, so on December 23, 1998, my thyroid and a few lymph nodes were removed. I was told I had 5-10 years. My calcitonin went down to 100.

In 2005 the calcitonin went up, and Mayo removed eight more nodes on the right side. In 2008 the calcitonin was higher again, and surgery at Mayo Clinic removed another 18 nodes, 12 of which were cancerous. In 2014 the surgeon removed a large palpable (sore) node from the right side.

At this point, my calcitonin is rising rapidly so I will have blood drawn and the sample sent to Mayo in Rochester. I've also written to the oncologist and endocrinologist at Mayo to schedule another follow-up appointment.

It has been 17 years since diagnosis. I feel the excellent care I received at Mayo Clinic saved my life. I will be 77 in June.

It is important for anyone diagnosed with MTC to seek experts in the disease.

My big question has been, "How did I get this type of cancer?" I can only guess, but I was exposed to lots of radiation, dental, etc., while serving in the Air Force. On a KB-29 flight crew in the Pacific in 1958-59, we were required to wear radiation detectors in areas of A-bomb testing!

A couple of years ago, I donated blood samples for Dr. Ryder, a Mayo endocrinologist who is conducting an in-depth study on MTC and its possible cure.

The sad part of this story is that in going from Michigan to Minnesota, I am "out of network" with my Blue Care insurance. The co-pay is a bit expensive. In addition, the expense of long distance transportation, lodging, etc. prevents many from seeking the care they need, since many medical facilities don't offer treatment to those with MTC. "Out of Network" should be outlawed!

My Own Roller Coaster Ride

By Jan Hofer

People say, "Boy! If I were to get cancer, I would want to get *your* kind. It's the *good* one to have".

Hello! I'm sorry; can you tell me what's *good* about it? Cancer is cancer; some are more aggressive than others, some are more treatable than others, some are common, some are rare, but bottom line, it's all still cancer with all the same fears and an end-game of death.

I can still remember the night my girlfriend was the one who told me I had cancer because my doctor's bedside manners were so bad that he couldn't tell me face-to-face. I think no matter the cancer, we all go through a few of the same steps/stages. First, we are in shock, this isn't supposed to happen to me, just other people. Then we are numb and are guided by our doctors in the path that *they* feel is the right way for us to go. Then we go through our denial stage, which also starts when we're saying this isn't supposed to happen to me. And don't forget our angry stage, again this wasn't supposed to happen to me, so how could God do this to me. I have so much going on in my life; I don't have time to deal with any more pressures. What was He thinking? Then after we come back to earth and get our feet a little settled in the ground we start to think things through. Maybe I should start to do some research on my own? Maybe there are other avenues that I can take with this. Or not. I do know of a few people who do just follow the path that their doctor decides for them. I guess I'm too much of a Doubting Thomas to have full faith in any doctor anymore these days…especially since Obamacare, but I won't go there! I want to play an active role in the "team" of decision making for what we are going to do next, what Plan B will be if Plan A doesn't work and, in the planning for the end, done my way, with dignity. Bottom line, it's my life and therefore ultimately it's my decision.

I am also *very* happy for others and my friends who have gotten cancers where they will see the days of being in remission. Remission, what is that??!! When you are misdiagnosed at the beginning of this journey, your outcome can be very different from one who is diagnosed correctly from the start. Your outcome can also be different by the timing of your diagnosis, if they found it early or if it's been growing in you for years before it's found. Then there is also the treatment path. Some of us have been told it's surgery or you're shit out of luck. MTC patients are just starting to see the beginning of what "treatment" options we could have coming up, if we make it that long. Did you know that if you call NCI and ask for a protocol for Medullary Thyroid Carcinoma you will be told they don't have one, at least that's what I was told in 1988. If you dare to ask why not (like I did), you will be told that the outcome isn't very good for that cancer and it would make their numbers look bad, therefore, there is no protocol. MTC patients also hear that we do not have the volume of people that is needed to do research; therefore our requests for grants to do research are denied. Now isn't that just sweet! I guess that makes us expendable.

It may be considered nice, lucky to have a slow growing cancer, which I guess is how some consider it to be a "good" cancer. BUT do you have any idea what it's like to live through a "Watch and Wait" for this cancer? You can be watching and waiting for *years*. Then they tell you but don't stress over this because stress just weakens the immune system, which can cause the cancer to grow. Yeah right, you tell me how to *not* stress when they are drawing blood from you every 6 months, running scans on you at least once a year if not every 6 months looking for this cancer so they can operate so you can just start the whole process all over again! You go in for imaging and the reception says, "Good luck, I hope they don't find anything." They look at you like you're the crazy one when you respond with, "Oh, but I hope they *do* find something, at least *then* I'll know where it's growing!" While I am talking about stress, there is a good book out there that has a "number" for the stresses in our lives and if you add all your stresses up you can see how it could give you cancer. The name of the book is *"Getting Well Again"* by Dr. O Carl Simonton, Stephanie Matthews-Simonton, and James Creighton. You can find the chart in Chapter 4: The Link Between Stress and Illness.

Another thing we Meddies deal with is that the doctors will start looking again or "watching" again once our numbers have doubled. I don't know of any other cancer that patients deal with doubling time. Before my last surgery in 2007 I had made it 11 years since the prior surgery. It's now 7 years since my last surgery and I have just reached the doubling time so we are looking again to see if we can find it, hopefully it will come back still operable, I'm not ready for the shit out of luck stage. Even after all these years of being a survivor I still get stressed every 6 months wondering if it's back again or if I'm safe for another 6 months. When it does come back that we need to start looking again, I *still* have a meltdown and go into my depression stage. I allow myself to have a little pity party and then kick myself in the butt and tell myself to get back up and start again…there's too much positive in my life that I'm not willing to let go of.

I have done some reading over the years of dealing with MTC. I am a big supporter of Dr. Bernie S. Siegel who wrote books called *"Love, Medicine & Miracles"* and *"Peace, Love & Healing"*. People find things out about themselves that they never knew. Some people feel that having developed cancer has also given them the right to now be able to tell someone *"no"*, they are not going to do something that they really didn't want to do in the first place. But before cancer, they never would have stood up for themselves and said so. They are able to move on from the shock, numb, angry, denial stages and still lead a productive life. Dr. Siegel also promotes the concept of a patient becoming a proactive part in their care. That's what I wanted, I didn't want people feeling sorry for me because I had cancer, and I still just wanted to be me. I also wanted to be completely involved in all the decision making of how or what treatment we were going to do. It takes a lot of research but in the long run it is so worth it. I truly believe that if I had not searched out three different ways to do my liver surgery, I would have already passed instead of just having to deal with a couple PE's (blood clots) in my lungs.

And then there are your friends. *Boy*, do you find out who they really are; not as many as you thought. After my total thyroidectomy surgery in February of 1988, I went back to work and I had lost all of my so-called friends accept for one or two. Coincidentally, one of them now also has another rare form of cancer and remarks to me how she also has lost most of her friends. Maybe it's the fear of not knowing what to say to a person when they are diagnosed. But you know what, even just saying that vs. turning and walking away from you is a lot more acceptable. This brings up another book I read called *"From Victim to Victor"* by a Dr. Harold H. Benjamin. In the section under *Being a Patient Active* they talk about friends or lack of after being diagnosed and how people don't know what to say to you. There's this statement, *"Other cancer patients have gone through what you are going through, so they can relate to you. Friends, however much they love you, can't relate to your struggle. They offer you sympathy without understanding, which is better than nothing, but people, particularly people with cancer, need to be understood."* I went to a support group for a while but I guess my stubborn Dutch attitude came through too strong and I just couldn't go any longer. It was a woman's group because at the time, they didn't know where to stick me. I would listen to one woman complain that her husband was not being supportive to her and now he has 3 jobs to keep him out of the house so he doesn't have to see or deal with her. She is the same woman who said if she shopped for clothes she would make sure her daughter liked them so when she was gone, her daughter could get use out of them. She is also the woman who said she even sleeps with her wig on because her husband doesn't want to see her bald head. My God woman, stand up for yourself! Another one said she was ready to die because that was God's plan for her. Really? I was always under the impression that God helps those who help themselves, not those who are just ready to lie down and die. I just don't understand how some people can just "accept" cancer like a prison sentence. I'm sorry, folks, but *this* girl is not going down without a damn good fight! Life has taken me through hell and back on this journey and I'm not done with the ride yet. I have made it through a divorce, now in a wonderful marriage, lost both my parents to colon cancer, have had both my hips replaced, and even a heart oblation procedure for SVT (supra ventricular tyachardia) and I'm not done with my journey yet. BUT I have been here long enough to see things I would have hated to miss that are so dear to my heart: meeting the true love of my life, my children's grammar school graduations, their high school graduations, one college graduation, seeing three grandchildren be born and being able to help raise them off and on. I may not be liked by some people (and my doctors think I'm a pain in the ass) but I have got one hell of a stubborn, strong-willed attitude towards this journey I'm on and as long as I'm still here kicking and fighting the whole way, I'm going to enjoy the ride until the end!

I currently have a "hobby farm" with calves to bottle feed every morning, the baby chicks are out of the bathtub and doing well in the brooder's coop, the ducklings have now also moved from the bathtub to their brooder's coop with a playground and kiddie pool. I collect eggs from the older chickens and ducks and make sure the older cows have grain, hay and alfalfa. When it's the season you can find me spending days at the kitchen table doing canning of many items like: applesauce, green beans, carrots, pumpkin, squash, and a variety of tomato items. I am trying to make cancer just a bump in the road.

The Dissection Of Thoughts

By Laura Druţău

Related to my experience with medullary thyroid carcinoma, I would like to share three stories.

The first about my father, whom I feel the duty to raise a homage to, the other about me and cancer, and the third about my doctor, the one who saved me in many ways.

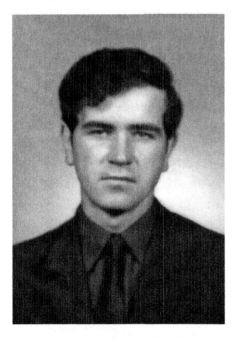

This is my father. His name was Vasile and he was a Captain in Police, after graduating. He was also on the Faculty of Law, in Cluj-Napoca, Romania.

He died at 40 years, in 1991. I was one year old then. He had symptoms of a pheochromocytoma many years before, but no one found his true disease. His symptoms were worsening and he started to talk more and more often about death. My mother thought he was joking, because he was a young, tall and strong man. But he felt something was not right with him. He told many times to my mother, "You will see, you will see".

All doctors gave him calcium and vitamins. He had also a small lump in the back (over the kidney). He asked my mother to massage it, and maybe it will pass. It was a pheochromocytoma, but nobody knew. He didn't tell the doctors about the mass in the back. He was a captain, and he was too proud to show his sickness, because he was well-known in the city.

One night, he felt very sick and my mother took him to the emergency room. He died 30 minutes after arriving. No time for goodbyes, no time for anything else. My mother wasn't next to him when he died, because the doctors tried to resuscitate him. They gave him shocks until they realized he would not come back to life anymore.

The autopsy diagnosis was pulmonary edema due to heart failure. His heart was very enlarged and the muscle of the heart very lax (only now, after 21 years, we realized it was because of an undiagnosed pheochromocytoma).

We lived with the idea he had only heart problems, like other men have.

Twenty-one years after his death I found my MTC and pheochromocytoma, my MEN2A mutation being finally confirmed. My two sisters and my mother do not carry the mutation. But my grandmother (the mother of my dad) died with the same symptoms at age 40.

My dad never knew he had MEN2A. He died leaving three kids behind (1, 7, and 10 years old). I was a baby and I do not remember him. Not even a memory in my mind. Only a few black and white pictures I have left, and a mutation that I inherited. Both the pictures and my MEN2A remind me of him often, in some kind of way. My mother never married again after his death, and I feel she could never pass over this loss.

The thing I want to expose with this story, is that an undiagnosed pheochromocytoma is not only undiagnosed to the one who has it. But it is also undiagnosed for the ones who suffer in many ways: after the passing of that person, or, without knowing they are lost on the same road, blurred by the same symptoms, without help.

The second story is about me.

If I should split my life in two big chapters, they would be: Life before MTC, and Life after MTC.

I found out I had cancer when I was 22 years old, after 3 years of knocking on all doors, to find out what's wrong with me. In the end, I had two surgeries, after one of them I woke up at the Intensive Therapy Unit, believing I was dead (as the anesthesia passed slowly, I could only hear, without moving, feeling anything, or opening my eyes). The right adrenalectomy was very painful for me. The second surgery came one week after. The recoveries were slow, and it was difficult to look at my own body, with so many scars. I hadn't known that they would become as common as going to the dentist.

When I went out from the hospital I was somehow happy, but when I arrived home I felt completely lost. I know it happens to some patients. I felt lost and I did not know how to start again. Where to begin? What makes sense anymore, and what does not? Why it happened? How long will I live? What should I do in the time remaining? How could I live that time better? What does it mean to really live fully? What is life? What comes after death? What is death? What is the sense of everything? What's the meaning of life? Why I didn't get any concrete treatment after surgery? Will I die sooner than I think? How should I tell to my mother that I will die? Will the worms eat me? Does a soul really weigh 21 grams, as they say? Why? Where did I come from? Where will I go? What is the truth? Where can I find it?

I was operated on January 2012, in a very cold winter. I remember the white snow, falling as in the stories. I remember the silence and the windy lonely ground.

I had a strong sensation of cold after my thyroidectomy, and the snow was even colder than I ever felt it before. The white landscapes of the city were the exact expression for the white emptiness in my soul. I felt completely alone in the world. I had never felt more lonely than those days.

After arriving home, I spent a few days staring at the empty walls, and looking out the window. I was staring many times at the stars, wondering what is out there. When I started to go for some walks in the city, I felt lost. Everything seemed estranged. In the end, I understood everything was the same, but *I* am now different. I was looking at all the people, things and places around me, wondering if I will still be there in one, two, five years.

As I stepped upon the freshly fallen snow, I was hearing the sound of that snow under my feet, realizing that I'm alive. Those were the short moments when I felt alive, back then.

After a few months I slowly put my forces together, and I decided that I have to understand what kills me, even if I have to die. I felt that it's a kind of responsibility to understand this world before leaving it. And on the other hand, if meanwhile I could help other people, that won't be a lost time on Earth. But to explain this decision, I have to pass to the third story, and talk about my doctor.

The third story is about a very calm man, whose name is Dan.

Dan was the doctor who saved my life in many ways, and maybe some of them I do not even understand yet. In the hospital, he, a surgeon of 35 years old (back then), became my best friend. My mother did not know anything about my two surgeries, because I tried to protect her from the worries. My sister stayed with me, as much as she could. And she was a huge supporter. But Dan was the stranger I needed, to recalculate all my life.

Dan made me open myself for the first time. I never used to talk about my feelings before him. Most of the time I tried to hide them, not to appear too sensitive, or exposed. I may have been a difficult patient making a lot of jokes to keep him at a distance from me, but he insisted that he stay and talk to me for hours, many days. I didn't realized the moment when he really caught me in his trap, but after my neck, he dissected all my thoughts. As days passed, after the hospitalization, we remained friends. To resume all our discussions in these years after the surgery, I would say he distracted my attention from death, to life.

The reason I say he saved me in many ways is because after he did my surgeries (together with his professor), he remained always near. Not too close, not too far. He made me change everything in my life. He gave me the desire to live again, to start again. I changed the pathway, from the Faculty of Arts to the Faculty of Medicine. I broke up with the boyfriend I had, I moved from the city I was living in at that time. I made other plans, and a new "life sketch" in my head. He kept telling me that everything is possible, and nothing is truly compulsory in life. He gave me the freedom, he gave me the wings to fly. Always supporting me from a distance, in a silent way.

Dan is the special person I met, that changed my path forever, and gave me the strength to go on.

In the end, I want to write a few things about this type of cancer. There is a book called "Staring at the Sun", written by Irvin Yalom. It helped me a lot during my post-hospitalization weeks. The book says there are two things that you can't look straight to: the sun, and the death. Even if both presences are there all our days during life.

The sad part of the fact that a young person has MTC is obvious, it's difficult to build a life in the presence of a silent cancer which may not kill you, but neither does it let you live carefree.

The positive part of this story, is the power this MTC gave me. It is not being afraid of anything, anymore. And to look straight to the sun, as Yalom says. If you feel your life is a bonus time, then you are not afraid of losing it anymore. That gives you the immense power and courage to do all the things you would be afraid to do. That gives you the infinite capacity to confront anything. To try, to risk, to insist, to do more.

Medullary Thyroid Cancer/ MEN 2a, A Daughter's Story

By Christine S.

Five years. Wow! This summer will be the 5th anniversary of my thyroidectomy and the surgeries for 2 of my 3 children. How can time go so slowly, and so fast, at the same time? What a roller coaster that year was after my mom's diagnosis. Everything was happening so fast. Waiting for test results was so slow. My mom had her surgery late in 2009. Then all of a sudden, we knew that the cancer she was diagnosed with could be hereditary. I know that doctors don't want us to do research on the Internet. It can be helpful, and it can be terrifying. Probably mostly terrifying. When it was confirmed that mom's cancer was hereditary, I jumped into action with my own testing and appointments. I was so worried that it was positive. I *so* wanted to spare the kids any worry or surgeries for them. My genetic test went out to a different lab than the rest of my family's tests, since I live in another state, and it took a while for my results. My calcitonin was 295. I can remember that clearly. I also clearly remember my primary care doctor telling me that she has never had a case of MTC and had only heard of it in medical school, but she referred me to the genetic counselor and surgeons.

Once I got my results back, I had to tell the kids that they now needed to be tested, too. From the research that I had done, I knew that time was of the essence in getting the thyroid removed to try and prevent the cancer. I had been working on getting referrals set up so that as soon as I got the results, I could make their appointments for their testing. My youngest daughter was only 9 at the time. Once I told them and they started their own testing, she was very anxious and scared about the possibility of needing the surgery. I did not know how to manage her fear. I had my own fear that I had to keep under control. I was worried about my mom, my two brothers, a niece, 3 nephews, my three kids and myself. Waiting for test results was excruciating. I know how devastated my mom was for each new positive result. She was heartbroken. But we had to be strong and deal with it head-on.

When talking to my own kids, I have always tried to give my kids the truth and not try to sugar coat things. They deserve respect and information. They are very smart, insightful kids and I probably wouldn't have been able to hide much anyway, they would have seen through it. So, it's best to tell them the truth about the importance of getting testing/surgery ASAP. They needed to understand the importance of being proactive and taking control to get testing, surgery and now long-term follow-up. The hard part was containing my own fear while also trying to project strength and calmness. I had to show I had things under control and I was doing whatever I could to take care of them and protect them. I had to follow their lead when discussing the diagnosis and answering their questions about the surgery. The hospital where their surgeries were performed (on the same day, only about a month after mine) gave them a tour of the floor and the activity room, the hospital rooms, etc. to help them know what to expect on the actual day and to help ease their fears and concerns. I don't know if all hospitals do that, but it was appreciated in this case.

One thing that I didn't expect was having to deal with my oldest daughter's concern for her brother and sister and her guilt for *not* having to have the surgery. She wondered why she was spared. She knew how scared her little sister was and felt horrible that her sister had to go through it and she didn't. She wished it would have been her, because she felt that since she was a few years older, she could have handled it better. My son didn't really talk about it at all. He just accepted it and wanted to move on afterwards, as fast as possible. He had to stay an extra day in the hospital due to low calcium, but after that he was ready to get home. They both recovered well from the surgery. My calcitonin dropped and has been reported as <5 since after surgery. My pathology showed that I had MTC in both sides of the thyroid but the lymph nodes they took were negative. Both of the kids' pathologies were negative, which is lucky considering that their ages were already at or over the recommended age limit for having a thyroidectomy. Now, after 5 years their scars are hardly visible, while mine is still more noticeable. I don't really care about my scar. It's just another battle wound, and I am still here, as are my kids. They are strong, have grown like weeds (I'll soon be the shortest in the house, and I'm 5'8"!), and are smart, funny, ornery teenagers. They are good about taking their meds, but even after so much time, I still ask regularly. I guess it's just me being the mom. As of right now, we have annual follow up appointments with the endocrinologist for blood work and medication levels. I am so thankful that we knew about this cancer early on for them and I am looking forward to them having long, productive, happy lives.

MTC: A Sister's Journey

By Lisa Leesman

My 49-year old brother was diagnosed with MTC in August 2012. His initial surgery, a total thyroidectomy (TT) was done by his ENT in Florida after she discovered a nodule during a routine visit for sinus trouble. When the biopsy came back medullary thyroid cancer (MTC), he needed help going forward, and that's when I became involved and went into action, becoming his advocate.

It's amazing how much good information is available on the Internet if you stick to reliable sites. I started out knowing absolutely nothing about MTC, but quickly got up to speed. I suggested a few Centers of Excellence for his follow-up surgery, and he selected Memorial Sloan-Kettering due to its reputation and location close to the entire extended family. Since he lives alone, we wanted him to be able to stay with family during his recovery.

Shortly after his initial diagnosis, I joined the MTC Facebook group and have educated myself about this disease so I can help him in the future. I'm the kind of person who likes to be informed, to be able to react without surprise when things happen. I read each MTC Facebook entry in depth every day. I cry when an MTC patient dies, I cringe when I see surgical photos, I pray for all the sick and their caregivers, and I do it so I am prepared to help him and myself as his disease progresses.

My brother has opted not to join the MTC Facebook group, and doesn't read much on MTC. Everyone deals with cancer in his or her own way. I devour information in advance. He has to deal with it as it comes, in pieces.

I accompany my brother to New York City (250 miles from my home) for nearly every medical appointment. We fly in and out of NYC from our separate hometowns, meeting at the airport or the hotel, and navigate our way through the appointments together. I take copious notes and e-mail them to him after each appointment. I keep a three-ring binder with all the e-mails and background information on this disease. I carefully observe the other cancer patients in the waiting rooms at Sloan-Kettering and wonder what's next for him. He doesn't seem to notice the other patients.

Between appointments, especially when his blood work comes back showing a rise in his calcitonin and CEA, he phones me and needs to be reassured. I read my notes back to him, quoting his doctors, reminding him of what we were told to expect. It's a huge help to have these notes. It allows me to reassure him while giving him correct information right from the doctor's mouth.

Regretfully, I had had almost no contact with my brother for nearly a decade before his diagnosis. We lived in different states, even different continents for a time. Things were said and done that created a deep rift. But with the MTC diagnosis, everything changed in an instant. Past hurts were forgiven. We only look forward now. Crises have a way of doing that.

It's The Small Things In Life That Count

By Mary Ann

In August of 1999, I was in the shower and soaping up when I felt a lump on the left side of my neck. I thought to myself, "Hmm". I felt around a bit and everything seemed the same on both sides. I went on with my day.

I worked at a very large medical practice at that time and I asked one of the doctors to feel my neck. She said she wanted me to have an ultrasound because she thought I had a simple cyst. A couple of weeks later I went for my ultrasound. The technician did the test and then went and got one of the radiologists. He repeated the ultrasound, looked at me and said, "You have *cancer*. You need to see your PCP immediately!"

Talk about freaking out! My heart started racing, and I was sweating with all these confusing thoughts and images running through my mind at supersonic speed. I went right up to the second floor where my PCP's office was located. I told his receptionist what had just happened and she got me an appointment for first thing in the morning, but not for two days, because my doctor was at a conference.

I went home in shock, and when I walked in, my fiancé asked me how the test went. I couldn't look at him or talk to him. I just kept busy looking everywhere but at him, and avoiding him. I knew that if I told him and he touched me that I would lose all control and break down into a heaping, blubbering mess. Finally, he stood up and pulled me into a hug and then asked me again what had happened. And I told him. Both of us were in shock, so we went out for a blast on his Harley to try to get me focused on something else.

I saw my PCP in two days. He felt my neck and made me swallow a few times with his hand on the front of my throat. He called the surgeon, and I went right over to his office. He did the same exam and ordered lab work and a biopsy with a radiologist.

My fiancé was in the room when they did the biopsy. It was SO painful, and you know you can't move. They put that needle in my neck three times, and each time was worse than the previous time. I had a huge bruise on the front of my neck, and all I could think of was that people would think someone had punched me.

Then the waiting began. I am not good at waiting. It was hell, the waiting. Finally, the surgeon called me and said it seemed I had a very rare form of cancer and that he wanted me to have a CT scan to see if it had spread beyond my thyroid gland. It hadn't, and surgery was scheduled for October 5, 1999. I still didn't realize I had cancer.

I had my surgery and I stayed overnight in the hospital. I didn't need any pain meds. Believe it or not, I wasn't in any pain, even though I had just had my neck sliced wide open. What I did remember was a really bad sore throat and the feeling that I had a golf ball stuck in my throat. I drank ginger ale all through the night and that made my throat feel better. The surgeon came in the next morning to discharge me, and he couldn't believe that I hadn't asked for pain meds.

Back then they didn't take out the lymph nodes, and I had labs for calcitonin done at regular intervals. Never saw an endocrinologist, so my PCP ordered the labs. The surgeon retired and that was that.

When I first heard that I had cancer, I felt like I took a punch to the gut. My mind was racing with a million thoughts. Am I going to die? What will happen to my kids? Who will take care of my elderly mother? I had just started a new life and that life was good. I didn't want it to end. I was so scared! After a while, I knew I had to do what I had to do. Had the tests, had the surgery, took the meds. Each time I had to have the calcitonin test, I would have such anxiety, hoping it would remain undetectable.

I knew I had a very rare cancer. *So* rare, that I didn't know a single person that had it. I had no one to talk to. No support groups like other cancers do. Then one day I found "our group". A wonderful group that has become family to me. There were others out there just like me! I now know what to expect from this beast we call MTC. I know what can be done about it. I am not scared and alone anymore.

After all these years, it doesn't scare me anymore. It makes me angry. So angry, that I will do whatever I have to so it doesn't consume me with that fear anymore. I am stronger now and I am a WARRIOR! We fight and we have a plan to conquer this beast.

My calcitonin was undetectable for years, and then it started increasing a bit. I got a bit nervous, but my new PCP didn't say anything. Finally, one day I asked him why he wasn't concerned. He replied, "Isn't Dr. X following you?" Dr. X was the endocrinologist in the practice. And I said I'd never seen her. He was astonished that someone with MTC wouldn't be followed by an endocrinologist. He got me in right away, and she did so many labs, it was unreal. She told me that the MTC was active again, and the room spun. I thought I was going to pass right out. I was moving from Massachusetts to Arizona in less than a month.

Fortunately, the new doctor I found here in Arizona referred me to a wonderful surgical oncologist, and he has been following me since. I did have a bilateral neck dissection in December of 2013, and all 64 nodes were negative for MTC.

Through all the MRI's of my abdomen I was showing that the disease had moved to my liver, and we're keeping an eye on that. My calcitonin and CEA levels continue to rise and I have seen an oncologist, too. No treatments yet. Not until we need to. We just keep going on, day by day.

MTC is not a good cancer by any means. It will never go away, but it makes you realize that it's the small things in life that count, not possessions. The family times. Watching your grandchildren play soccer, and having a holiday meal. Face time with loved ones who live across the country.

I love spending time in my garden, watching the hummingbirds and the butterflies. I still work full time, but someday I may not be able to. We'll cross that bridge when we come to it. But even though I have the terrible disease, life is good! I wouldn't trade my life for anything. I have the best husband, who has stood by me with all the craziness that comes with this beast.

My "meddie" family is the very best. We joke, love, support and grieve with each other. I thought I was all alone with this cancer because I didn't know one single soul who had it. But I have met many wonderful people through our support group. I wouldn't give them up for the world.

Eager To Live

By Becky Mack

In February of 2009, I was trying to live my young adult life. After receiving positive results for a genetic disorder that causes endocrine health issues and tumors, I found myself face to face with a doctor who was unsuccessfully trying not to cry. "It's Medullary," she said to me. "It's cancer. Very rare." One hour before that, I had been lying in a room, wearing nothing but a hospital gown, with huge needles jabbing my neck. I was freezing. The technician said, "I know it's difficult, but try to stay as still as possible. We're too close to your carotid artery." *Carotid artery? Who cares about my carotid artery? Why can't I just sit here and cry?*

"You'll probably live with this for the rest of your life," the oncologist told me. Through tears, I asked her, "Am I going to live to see 50?" She stopped, looked at me with concern and truth in her eyes, and said, "We can never answer questions like that definitively. We are going to take care of you."

I remember reading books that described moments that felt like the world had stopped. That's how I felt in that moment. I was breathing and moving, but I wasn't part of everything that was happening around me. But this wasn't a dream. It wasn't even a nightmare. This was my life. It was the truth. It was ludicrous, but absolutely legit at the same time. I was angry. *How can the world stand so still? How can MY world stop just as I'm about to sail?*

I called my Mom and listened to the shock that she tried to hide from her voice. Giving her that news was the scariest, saddest, most nauseating thing I've ever had to do. I'm an only child. If there's one thing I never want to re-experience in my life, it's the moment when I felt my head and my heart turned to watery tears as I said to my Mom, "I have cancer".

I spent about a month without sleeping for more than three or four hours a night. I barely ate and I worried into complete emptiness. A month of tests. Scan after scan, blood test after blood test, wait after wait.

The waiting. For almost a full month, I felt like all I did was wait, and wait some more. I questioned and I speculated. Was the cancer in my liver? My bones? My lungs? What stage was I? What was the prognosis? Would I have to get chemotherapy? Was this pain in my rib cage related to my cancer? Waiting sucked the soul out of me. I was drowning.

In 1999 my Father committed suicide, and ten years later I finally understood how it felt to yearn for the kind of sleep that could erase all my anxiousness and pain. Ten years later, in 2009, I yearned for a Dad that I never had because he was so engulfed in depression. One night I sat on the back patio of our small apartment in Texas and cried until my head throbbed and kicked the shit out of the wooden barrier that surrounded it. I hurt my bare foot so much that I didn't even care anymore. *I will die soon anyway.*

By August of 2009 my young adult life had been stolen from me and I was older than I ever expected to be at the age of 28. It would be a little more than six months from the date of my diagnosis before we had a plan. Those six months were undeniably the worst, most nightmarish six months of my life. I quit my job, stopped talking to almost everyone I knew and spent a lot of time inside my own mind, re-evaluating everything I'd ever done in my life. My undiagnosed genetic disorder had resulted in stage 4a Medullary Thyroid Cancer that had spread to distant lymph nodes in my neck. I would most likely never see it go away and I'd live with the effects of the genetic disorder forever.

The cancer was still measurable in my blood six months after an almost ten-hour neck surgery. I was being seen by one of the world's best medical teams at MD Anderson Cancer Center in Houston, Texas. I'd have to spend a good part of my life waiting. Watching and waiting to see what the cancer would do. More waiting. I had an oncologist now. I was 28, finishing my college degree, unemployed, and I had an oncologist. *I know that other people have done this cancer thing, so why can't I?*

"You are stable," my doctor said to me recently. "Go drink some beer, have fun. Enjoy your life." I am 34 years old, pretty close to turning 35. I'm a young adult living with an incurable form of cancer. I'd like to see 55, 65 and 75. I don't want to die. I'll never be the person I was, what felt like 100 years ago.

Some people say a survivor is someone who's brave in the face of cancer, someone who takes things on head first without breaking down. Some people say that having cancer makes you some sort of a hero or an inspiration, that you're fighting or battling, and you either win or lose.

I disagree. No one loses. I don't think I'm fighting, and I'm not a hero. I'm just surviving my life.

I'm trying to maneuver through each day the best way I know how. Sometimes that means I cry or break down. Sometimes that means I get pissed off when people judge me or roll their eyes at me when I'm talking about my cancer. "She's always looking for attention," I've heard. "She's fine. Look at her." Sometimes that means I'm irritated when people look at my full head of hair and diminish my cancer experience. Sometimes that means that being brave or putting a smile on my face is not an option because I'm really scared and I don't have all the answers. I'm just trying to stay afloat, and I think that's okay.

I'm not sure how to end my part in this book, this memoir. Through tears, all I can think of is what I've learned in the past six years, what I've lived and how panic has drowned me in the process of trying to find what's normal. I could never sum up what I've discovered about myself and the people around me in a paragraph, a page or even a book.

I've learned the art of waiting, and how to gently explain my test results to my Mom. I've learned how to take notes when I'm talking to the doctor and to fire doctors who make me feel uncomfortable, or like a burden. I've learned that "tomorrow is never promised" is not some cliché, it's the truth. I've learned that running helps me figure stuff out, panic is okay, and normal doesn't exist. My cancer can grow or change at any time, and it's acceptable to talk about it. It's ok to speak my mind. What is unacceptable is not telling my story when I know children with MTC who may not see the age of 30. If I want to do something in my life, I need to do it NOW. I had to learn that if you don't face something, it doesn't go away. It just lingers somewhere in the hidden parts of your soul.

Cancer is a cluster fuck. It's a turbulent, unrelenting piece of my life that I'm forced to set aside when I go to work every day. Cancer makes me wait, and wait some more. It's a reminder that I'm my Mother's only child and I never want to let my disease break her heart. I loathe it.

What's more important than my hatred of cancer is my love of living. Every morning I wake up eager to live. Every day I tell my cancer story to anyone who's willing to listen. Every moment is a chance to help someone who wants to go to sleep forever and deserves a desire to live. I think I've forever exhausted enough time trying to chase the moon and demanding answers for things that might just be unanswerable. I think I've wasted enough energy speculating and wondering with what-ifs. That much effort crushes the soul. I feel like I have a good foundation, even if my thoughts aren't in the same place as most of the people with whom I interact every day. My voice is strong and my efforts are focused and meaningful. I might die one day because of my cancer, and I might not. I might have to get chemotherapy one day and I might not. But if and when those things become a part of my life, I'll run it out, talk it out, and remember that what matters the most isn't chemotherapy or death.

It's telling my story and what happens in between.

Diane's Story

By Diane Saxon

(Editor's note: The first entry here was from Diane to Myrtle Young. The second was written by Diane's son, Mike.)

Myrtle, thank you so much for your kind words. I am hanging in there. I will be relieved once we find out what is causing the pain. I have had this cancer for so long with no pain, it worries me that it's now hurting.

I sent my local CT scans to Dr. Gramza on Monday. She compared them to my November scans at NIH. Dr. Gramza said she couldn't see much of a difference meaning... it may not be my liver...which is what my local hospital told me it was...this could be good news. (It would also mean that the Ponatinib is working.) It could be the MTC spreading to my ribs, which from what I hear, is painful. It sounds crazy, but I prefer it be my ribs, even though MTC has not spread to my bones, yet. This is because my ribs could be more treatable than my liver...I think. Dr. Gramza is going to be ordering more scans when I am there next week so I should know more then.

I am a fighter and have a lot of faith in God. He has helped me through this for 34 years now...and I believe he will help me now. So many more of our friends have had harder struggles than I, example... Bill, Julie, Rob, Dave, Jim, and more. They will have a setback and then bounce back...I'm so amazed and inspired...

Thank you again for you kind words. With love, Diane

From Sonia Prud'homme:

Mike, Diane Saxon's son, posted a tribute for his mom on her personal site today. He agreed to share it with the group. So here is a beautiful tribute to his mom and our meddie friend, Diane:

Remembering Mom

Mom was many things to the people in her life:
Grandmother
Mother
Wife
Sister
Aunt
Friend
Hot Dog Marksman
Teacher
Role model
Inspiration
Hero
Fighter
Survivor

And she was all of those things before her sickness came back in 2009.

Mom was kind and compassionate, yet strong and resolute. Always putting the welfare and happiness of others before her own, she was the most caring individual I've ever met. Even in her last weeks, the impact on her family and the other brave warriors fighting the sickness of her declining health was among the top of her concerns.

Throughout my life, from as far back as I can remember, Mom made special efforts to have quality time with me, sharing her interests and engaging in mine. Whether we were typing in programs on the family computer to see what they would do, rescuing Zelda, taking on the Mother Brain, watching our favorite shows, playing our board games, saving Krondor, vanquishing Xeen, listening to the same music, taking pictures together, or any of the other many activities that we enjoyed together, Mom always made time to spend with me.

When I was growing up, we moved around a good bit, as do many military families. Regardless where we were, whether we spoke the local language, and how homesick she was, Mom always made sure that everything felt normal, stable, and consistent. Home was always where we were.

Mom taught me that parenting is just as much about the time spent together as friends doing the same thing as it is the formal parent-child relationship that my friends' parents had with them, and that always showed in how my friends loved my mom and usually wanted to come over to our house. That is an example I am trying very much to follow.

Mom taught me about respecting myself and others and that to win respect, you have to offer it first. She taught me to treat everyone as I want to be treated. She taught me responsibility and that, in her words, "Do the right thing, and things will usually work out for you." I live by those words to this day.

I've always heard that you learn how to have relationships by watching how your parents get along. My parents were best friends, and the mutual love and respect between them has shown through in everything that they did for at least my lifetime. I am very grateful to have grown up in that atmosphere with my parents as role models, having the most loving and balanced marriage that I've seen. Steph and I have modeled a great deal of our ideal of marriage on Mom and Dad's, as have others.

Of the many things that I have to be thankful for, one of the most prominent is the relationship between my daughter, Natalia, and Mom. In January of 2008, Steph and I were blessed with our daughter, Natalia. From the first video call, to the first time they met in person, for most days over the following six years, and until mom's final few days, Mom lit up, her eyes sparkled, and regardless how she was feeling or what else was going on with the world, she would smile as if she were falling in love all over again.

I am very grateful that Natalia was able to have that relationship with Mom and that they got as much quality time together as they did.

Mom fought with her sickness for 34 years, but she did not let it define who she was. She was an inspiration to those around her, especially those fighting the same fight. Mom made the best of every situation presented to her, choosing to look at the bright side, and maybe even laugh a little, no matter the situation.

I am very honored and proud to be her son.

Rest in peace, Mom.

I love you.

Bound Me Now To The Soil

By T. F. Tritt

Bound me now to the soil,
Let treasures rich grow with toil.
My arms, my legs, my back shall ache,
This, my life, ere I make.

Cast me now against my sin
Tearing part in soulless wind.
When I die, when I wake,
This, my life, ere I fake.

Cold fury, winter's hearth,
Scouring flames tear apart.
My mind doth yearn, my soul forsake,
This, my life, ere I rake.

All thought, drowning deep,
Peace and calm all I keep.
Surface churns, ripples break,
This, my life, ere I take.

In my heart a dream of peace,
In my hand an ivory wreath.
Either one is mine to take,
This, my life, ere I wake.

Life Is Good And My Journey Continues

By Jan Hofer

Life before the Journey

You think you've got it all, and everything's going to be just fine. I was married and had two beautiful children, one boy and one girl. Life was good. Then as the years of marriage moved on we grew in separate directions instead of in the same direction. His self-esteem was getting worse, and me? Well, I was just doing what I knew had to be done to make ends meet. For me that meant having to give up being a stay-at-home mom and go back into the work world. I remember one of my job interviews where the manager asked me, "So, if you've been at home with children for the last 2-3 years, what makes you think you can still type?" I looked at him as I picked up my things and said, "I guess for the same reason that once you've learned how to ride a bike you never forget."

I landed a great job, starting off part time, which turned into a full time position within the first year. In fact, I proved I was able to jump back into the work force when my manager put me in charge of running a "light duty" work crew to put together First Time Rider's Kits for our local bus system. I did that job well enough that when she changed companies she took me with her. I'd say that calls for a small pat on the back. Kudos to you, girl!

So as I said, life was good. I told my best friend, "Something is going to have to happen to turn my marriage around, a life-or-death situation." Little did I know that within months those words would come true.

Suspicious "Marble"

I'd been having diarrhea issues and talked it over with my primary care physician (PCP), who diagnosed lactose intolerance since the episodes seemed to be related to my consuming dairy products. I also told him about my "pet marble" (lump in the upper left side) in my neck. He brushed me off and said it was probably just a swollen gland and to call him if it was still there in six months.

However, before that time was up I had to call him from work and tell him that I had a *really* strange situation. I had to pull the cartilage out in my throat so it could fall back down into place, and it really hurt putting it back. He again blew me off and said, knowing you, you were laughing too much. Call me if it happens again.

Then I had my six-month dental checkup and the dentists had just started doing the cervical gland checks. My dentist did the check and then turned to write notes. Being the smart-ass that I am, I asked him, "Oh, come on, John (as I held my button front shirt open at the neck), aren't you gonna feel any further?" Then I added, "I thought you'd want to feel my pet marble." Well *that* got his attention. He rolled back over and asked where my pet marble was and felt all around it. He looked at me and said, "You will go to a specialist by the end of this week or I'll take you!"

So off to an ENT I went. He felt around the pet marble, then started to ask questions. He had come to the conclusion that the birthmark mole on my backside just above my "crack" was responsible. He said this sort of birthmark tends to throw off benign, almond-shaped tumors, then added, "But let's go for an ultrasound to see what we're dealing with." This was 1987, the Thursday before Thanksgiving, and little did I know that this would be the start of a long journey for me.

The Beginning of My Journey

My first surgery was scheduled for January 1988. Insurance said why waste a full year of your deductible? Wait for the surgery until January to remove my "pet marble," which the doctor thought was nothing more than a calcium buildup on a lymph node. Surgery was a breeze. They did find a tumor, but didn't know the status of it yet. I returned to the ENT in 10 days to have my staples removed and he requested that I come into his office so we could talk. He was reading to me out of his medical book, and nothing was registering until he got to the end and talked about fatalities at one, five and 10 years. I said to him, "This sounds like some pretty serious shit." He came back with, "Young lady, you probably just saved your own life." He said I'd have to go back for a total thyroidectomy and removal of some lymph nodes in five weeks, after I healed from this biopsy surgery.

Horrible bedside manner. I left his office knowing I had a thyroid "disease," but not knowing it was cancer. My girlfriend called me that night to ask what I'd found out. I told her the same thing. "I've got a thyroid disease and have to go back for more surgery." She asked what it was and I said, "I don't know. Let me read it to you off my bill." Then she asked me if I had a dictionary in the house and I said yes. She said go get it and read about carcinoma and she would stay on the phone. *That* was the moment I found out. Around 7-8 p.m. I called dispatch and said I had a family emergency and send my husband home. He radioed dispatch and said he'd be home at the end of his shift at 2:00a.m. Gee, this should have been my first heads-up that there was nothing left to this marriage.

My parents came out for two weeks for the second surgery and to help with my children while I healed. The endocrinologist said there was a good chance this could be hereditary and my family should have a calcitonin blood test done. My father's response was, "No. If I gave this to you I don't want to know." I told him that his results could make a difference in how they would have to treat me. He still didn't care and said no.

After being diagnosed I took a serious look at my marriage and initiated counseling. Well, I did that three times in three separate years. I even moved to strengthen the family unit by buying a small motel that we could run as a family, but things still didn't improve. I had a third surgery to remove more lymph nodes, and once again it was my parents who came to help with my children and the motel. My husband wouldn't take any time to help. The final heads up about the marriage came with that surgery, when he told me to find a ride home from the hospital because he was too busy to come get me.

I had also read a few books to learn to cope with cancer. I kept reading about how once someone was diagnosed it gave them "permission" to start saying no to people, to finally do what they wanted in life instead of what other people expected of them, that it was okay to take control of your own life. It was time to make a tough decision, and I decided it was time to take care of me because no one else was going to do it for me. I made the choice to move out and back to Denver to take care of me. I was told I was being selfish, and my parents were more upset with what people would think of them having a "divorced" daughter versus what I was going through.

So once again I found myself in a "life goes on" situation. I struggled in and out of jobs and with trying to pay my own way. In addition, my husband had me pay for child support while he continually lied in court about his income, saying he made only $10K a year, and I was making more than he was.

I tried dating, but I was always upfront about my situation. I am a package deal and come with not only two wonderful children but also with cancer! Let me tell you, big boys *do* know how to run, and fast. It had been 4-5 years, and one weekend when I had my children, my daughter told the man I was dating, "You must have something my Mom likes because she's kept you around longer than three months." I've always told my children they needed to make a mental list of what they were looking for in a mate, and if who they were with didn't fit most of that bill, why waste their time keeping that person around? This man had almost everything on my mental list, and I did want him to stick around. One of the most impressive things about him was the fact that when I told him about my package deal, he said, "I don't care. It's you I love and it's all part of the package." To this day I still call him my guardian angel. We were married in February 1996.

I've gone through many things during this journey. My mother and father were both diagnosed and subsequently passed from colon cancer. I had a heart ablation (SVT) procedure done, and as of last year both hips have been replaced. I also had two big MTC surgeries with my second husband, who stood by me the whole time. Second surgery was a liver resection, and no one was expecting blood clots within 12 hours of surgery. They wanted to put me on a respirator but I said "no", so I was one of the first that they tried "the helmet" on, and it worked. To this day I deal with breathing problems due to the paralyzed vocal cord and the partially paralyzed diaphragm and have to be on oxygen at bedtime. But I watched both my children graduate from high school and one from college, have three beautiful grandchildren whom I get to see all the time, and a wonderful husband whom I wouldn't trade for the world. So once again, even with living with MTC almost half my life now, *life is good* and my journey continues.

Facebook Postings

By Julie Tavernier DiSanto

"Diagnosis one year ago today...hmmm... kind of strange, but feeling so much more blessed and appreciative of my life, my husband, my kids, my family, and my friends. Looking for the joy in my everyday moments...try it!! Xoxo"

"Ok...so just a little "funny" to share...in all my glorious baldness right now, when I look in the mirror, I can't help but see a little of my three handsome brothers looking back at me! Hysterical! (wink emoticon)"

God Is Greater Than Any Problem I Have

By Tom Joiner

In April 2010, a few months after my 48th birthday, I went to my local primary care doctor with symptoms of prolonged diarrhea and depression. I was told it was stress related, which could have been entirely possible considering I've been a small business owner since the age of 20.

Within the next two years I went six times to the same doctor, complaining of continued diarrhea, depression, weight loss and sleeping difficulties. In April 2011, he put me on antidepressant medication, which after three months showed no improvement. On March 15, 2012, I was also experiencing heavy sweating and had noticed a bump on my neck. A week later, blood work was performed, which indicated my testosterone and thyroid were normal. Two weeks later I visited the ER for extreme diarrhea. This doctor got very nervous once he saw the bump on my neck. A CT scan was performed a week later and the radiology doctor told me he saw a large abnormal mass in my neck area. He promptly scheduled an appointment with a local ENT, at which time a fine needle biopsy was performed. The biopsy report came back positive for cancer. I was then scheduled for a major needle biopsy to determine the type. At my next appointment on May 3, 2012, the ENT told me he thought it was anaplastic thyroid cancer and I probably had six months to live. I needed to "get my affairs in order." He told me surgery was not an option and that he would arrange for me to see a chemotherapy doctor, along with a radiology doctor the following week.

The next day, May 4, 2012, I requested my medical records from that local ENT doctor, who, surprisingly enough, questioned why I was seeking a second opinion! My father then called his primary doctor, whom I had personally met, to discuss my situation, and that doctor said to go to the Mayo Clinic in Rochester, Minnesota.

The following day, Saturday, we applied online to Mayo, and without having heard back from them (they're not open on weekends), I left on Sunday, May 6, 2012, for the Mayo Clinic. It was about a 10-hour car ride from Grand Haven, Michigan. About three-fourth into the trip I received a call from the Clinic setting me up for an appointment on June 5th. I felt very disappointed at having to wait a month for my visit, and was in the process of turning around when I had another one of the many "God moments" that I was blessed with throughout this whole journey. I had a friend who was being treated at the Clinic at that time. We had originally planned to meet up once I got there so he could help me get acclimated to the Clinic and surrounding area. I made a call to him, explaining that I wouldn't be able to be there for another month, but he encouraged me to continue to the Clinic anyway and suggested there was a quicker way to be seen (they refer to this as a "checker" as I later found out). Within a day and a half of "signing in" I was called in to see my first Mayo doctor, an ENT. He reviewed the records I'd brought with me and immediately ordered a blood test. Within two hours I was back in his office, discussing the results. (I was, and continue to be, absolutely amazed at how efficiently and quickly the results are obtained.) The correct diagnosis was medullary thyroid cancer and the calcitonin level was 5,600. At this point I was confused because my local doctor had tested my thyroid through blood work and indicated it was normal. My Mayo ENT clarified this by saying that most local doctors are not familiar with medullary cancer because of its rarity, and therefore do not test for it.

They immediately scheduled me for surgery on May 29, 2012. The reason for the three-week delay was so the ENT surgeon could assemble the specific team of doctors necessary to be present at the surgery. At this point I was given ten days' worth of appointments to determine if I was healthy enough to undergo this extensive surgery. However, because I was a "checker" I was able to complete all tests within five days (and, more thanks to God, I was given the green light).

The subsequent surgery resulted in a bilateral TT, loss of a jugular vein, and loss of a nerve to one vocal cord, resulting in a raspy voice. Another surgery was performed on August 6th for some residual cancer found on my collarbone. To decrease the chances of reoccurrence, radiation was suggested, and subsequently performed six weeks later.

The first three weeks of radiation went very smoothly, with little or no side effects. The last three were somewhat difficult, but in my opinion, worthwhile. With the help of the American Cancer Society's Hope Lodge, located two blocks from Radiation Therapy at the Clinic, and their cheerful staff and volunteers, along with the many wonderful people I met there also going through chemotherapy and/or radiation, my stay was a time of emotional healing. The friendships I found there resulted in what became for me an extended family, some of whom I continue to maintain contact with today. The Hope Lodge is free for anyone going through chemotherapy and/or radiation for the patient and a caregiver (required).

After a year of continued visits and testing, while very happy to learn the cancer had not returned to my neck area, a few spots were detected in my liver, which resulted in a complicated cyroablation in January 2014. It was discovered that my airway for intubation was greatly restricted due to the surgeries and radiation. It was a very risky intubation as it turned out, but ultimately successful.

Then, in December 2014, after finding a few more spots in the liver, it was determined that either radiation or another ablation would need to be performed. However, due to my restricted airway, both doctors were reluctant to intubate due to an elevated risk of death. Things were looking pretty bleak at that point when, by the grace of God, we were approached in one of the skywalks at the Clinic by a doctor who thought we were lost (apparently we looked confused, which in this case, was a blessing). While chatting with him, he asked about my raspy voice, which prompted a few questions about how things were going during my visit there, etc. At this point, I mentioned "not well" due to the fact that both my doctors were uncomfortable with intubation, leaving me with limited choices. Right there in the hallway (and I tear up thinking about it), this doctor did a quick personal assessment of my airway and said he felt absolutely comfortable that, with his assistance, I could have a successful intubation, and indicated that we should let our doctor know that he was more than willing to help. As we found out later, this doctor is the head of the Anesthesiology Department, has been there for 30+ years, and did assist in the intubation. Both the intubation and the ablation were successful in December 2014. We consider this nothing short of a miracle!

My challenge continues, however, as recent visits have discovered a few new spots in my liver, which are too small to treat at this time, but God has blessed me in the past, and I feel confident He will be there for me through whatever comes up next.

While the past three years have been somewhat of a bumpy road, the positives have more than outweighed the negatives. Throughout my entire life I've known God. However I'm happy to say I'm *much closer* to Him now than I've ever been. I have felt God's absolute presence and strength, beginning with my decision to seek help at the Mayo Clinic, a much stronger and closer relationship with my family, a chance meeting with a significant other, Debbie, only three weeks before being diagnosed, who has been a major source of strength, determination and focus throughout the entire process, especially after having had to deal with her own Stage IV cancer nine years ago, and extending into significant closer relationships with my many friends. Hardly a day goes by where one or several of my friends hasn't stopped in or called to see how I'm doing. Countless family and friends have offered to accompany me on my trips to Mayo, and several have already made the trip.

While my family has always been somewhat close, we've gained an amazing amount of strength and togetherness through these challenges. I've always been a social person, but I have to say the number of people who have approached me upon hearing about my situation has far exceeded any in my pre-cancer days. While I've gained much knowledge in the cancer area through my own situations, I've been blessed to be able to help others through their struggles as well.

During free time at Rochester, and to help clear my mind, I was pleasantly surprised to find many interesting sites to see, some of which include the Plummer historical building, an absolutely gorgeous building located across the street from the Clinic, and which houses the 56 Carillon bells, one of the largest in the country, with the biggest bell topping out at 4 tons, the 40-room Mayowood Mansion, built by one of the Mayo brothers in 1911, the Plummer House, a 49-room mansion built by Dr. Plummer, who was considered a genius in his day and was very instrumental in many innovations still being used today at the Clinic, the St. Francis of Assisi Heights Spiritual Grounds, an amazing complex built to house 1200 sisters, the Soldiers Field Veterans Memorial, which honors Minnesota veterans who gave their life for our country, to name a few. I especially enjoyed the many opportunities for walking, either along the many miles of paved walkways along the Zumbro River (which I personally find very soothing), or through the 2½ miles of enclosed walkways from the Clinic to neighboring hotels, restaurants, shopping and other buildings, which is extremely nice in bad weather.

While waiting one day in a doctor's office, I happened to pick up a small daily devotional book to help pass the time. Ultimately, this book has become a daily necessity for me! I read it the first thing every morning, and find that it gives me wisdom and strength to help with my upcoming day.

I thank God first of all, and His amazing blessings, and also the knowledgeable, kind doctors and staff at the Mayo Clinic, the strong support and love from Debbie, my family, and my friends, for helping me navigate through these trying times.

God is Greater than any problem I have!

I Want To Be Well

By Christen Bordenkircher

"Do you want to be well?" It was a question that caught my heart off guard. As I prayed and quieted my spirit the night before my thyroid biopsy report came back, I sensed God ask me: *"Do you want to be well?"* Of course I do. That seems like a silly question. But the more I thought about this question... the same question that Jesus asked the man waiting for healing by the pool in the Book of John, chapter five, the more I realized that it was a valid question that my heart needed to answer with honesty. For the past two years, I had been feeling victimized by the difficulty of our life overseas. I had been feeling blindsided by medical issue after medical issue for each and every member of my family. I had been overwhelmed by the daily demands of figuring out what life looked like in a country where I was an outsider and was not fluent in the language, or the culture. But after sitting with this question for a while, my heart answered: *"Yes. I want to be well."* Wellness is a choice. Wellness is also an identity. Regardless of what my biopsy uncovered, I needed to not play the victim of any medical condition that I could face. I needed to choose to be well, physically yes, but also spiritually, emotionally, mentally, and relationally.

While making this choice to be well, I also was staying positive. Having a history of being overly nervous about physical symptoms, I've come to downplay the possibility of something going really wrong with my body. The doctors said it was unlikely to be malignant. It was. The doctors said it was most likely to be papillary thyroid cancer. It was the unlikely Medullary Thyroid Cancer. The surgeon said it was unlikely that it had spread to my lymph nodes. It had. What this 'unlikely' cancer has done has reminded me that you have to learn to expect the unexpected. You can't take anything for granted. And if it's unlikely, then you are probably within the norm.

I've never quite fit the mold of other people's expectations nor backed away from a life that is outside the norm of the American Dream. In September 2013, we moved to Turkey with our 2 year old son while 6 months pregnant with our daughter, who was due around Christmas. People made comments like: "You guys are brave" to which I'd respond, "Yeah, or really stupid." I mean, who quits their jobs, moves overseas just before adding a second child to the mix, and leaves behind a very successful private practice in counseling and photography business to start over in a new country? Apparently, we do.

From September 2013 to May 2015, we busied ourselves with language learning and helping a new counseling center get off the ground that would support the mental health of foreign aid workers living in the surrounding region. It was the craziest season of our lives and while we loved the people, the culture, the challenge of speaking in our new language, we also were living in a context where life takes more work and we had to navigate a system that we weren't familiar with or fluent in. We had one medical crisis after another, which left our friends and family back home with a compelling reason to keep checking in on us!

Our daughter was a terrible sleeper for over a year and our son struggled with anxiety at night, so it didn't seem unusual for me to struggle with extreme, chronic fatigue. But I was completely exhausted for those first two years. I'd get my kids to sleep around 8:30pm and then transfer to my bed for the night. I had no energy. Following my daughter's birth on New Years Eve, 2013, I also struggled with what I assumed was postpartum depression. This self-diagnosis was all I could do to make sense of fits of rage and moments of feeling utterly overwhelmed by daily life.

Many days, it just *felt like too much*. But we loved the people. We loved the work. We loved the opportunity to learn from a beautiful culture and group of people. Our commitment to these dreams of serving the people in that part of the world did not waver although my confidence in my own strength to persevere certainly was shaken from time to time.

In September 2014, we came home for a visit with family and friends as well as to have some medical work done. While back, I scheduled a visit with my general doctor in Michigan. It was a good visit as I shared my emotional struggles and fatigue. Right at the end of the appointment, my doctor did a quick thyroid check and said: *"You have an enlarged thyroid, we should keep an eye on that."*

We headed back to Turkey and began year #2 of life over the seas. We were optimistic and excited for this new year. We spoke some of the language. We had friends. We had a permanent apartment that we loved. Turkey had become home for us. We had fallen in love with the dear people around us and grown to appreciate the cultural differences. We were in a good place.

In January 2015, I contacted my doctor for some persistent nausea, lower left abdominal pain, fatigue, mood swings, and occasional headaches. She advised me to follow-up with doctors in our city to have my thyroid checked as well as see a GI specialist and get a full blood work-up done. But, I had two little kids under three years old. My time and energy were limited. A few months passed without me following up with a doctor.

In April 2015, my dear friend, Jennie, used her vacation time to come stay with us for a week at our home in our coastal city. She is an advanced nurse practitioner with a deep Christian faith. Before she came, she prayed with others that she could be an encouragement to us and also help us tackle some of our health stressors. We had a great time hosting her. One beautiful morning, we were sitting and drinking Turkish tea at a café along the Mediterranean. Once again, I was sharing our story of medical challenges and the rollercoaster of emotions that seemed to characterize my experience of life overseas. After sharing about my fatigue, mood swings, depression, and nighttime anxiety, she gently asked me,

"Actually, Christen, this may sound weird... but I've been looking at your thyroid and noticing that it seems a little enlarged. Would you mind if I check your thyroid."

She checked it. "Yep, you have a nodule." I asked her what it meant. She responded: "Well, it's most likely benign. It's quite common to have a nodule, but you should have it checked. Don't be surprised if they find more than one."

The following week, I found myself sitting in the office of a local ENT in our city. He felt the same nodule that my friend Jennie had found. I remember watching his face as he squinted in his eyes and I wondered if I could detect 'concern' or 'bad news' from the way in which he was reacting. He ordered an ultrasound on my thyroid and blood work. A few days later, I was lying down as an ultrasound tech was speaking in Turkish and finding five nodules. Two nodules were so large and strange looking that I had to keep telling myself that this was NOT a little baby growing inside me. But an ultrasound for a baby was way more exciting as you WANT to see growth and life. But for nodules, I knew this growth was undesired.

A biopsy was ordered on the 12mm and 22 mm nodules. It was *unlikely* that either of these would be malignant and this was just a precautionary measure. A week passed, and I finally got an email with my biopsy report, all in Turkish, since my doctor was away at a conference and I didn't want to wait for the results. It made no sense to my husband or me, so my husband set off on a mission to translate this medical document. We had someone help us translate it. We sent it to our nurse friend Jennie who doesn't speak any Turkish but we were desperate to understand the results of my biopsy. Here is what she emailed us:

"Christen, I've poured over the path report, and there are two words that jump out at me: follicular neoplasm. I think that's what was translated for you as a thyroid tumor, and unclear whether benign or cancerous? My friend, in my mind that is a term for thyroid cancer, i.e. thyroid follicular cancer - very, very treatable. It is true that "neoplasm" means tumor, or "new growth", and can be benign or cancerous, but when you add it to the term "follicular", it very likely refers to cancer. So if I've got the translation right, #1 is follicular neoplasm/suspect follicular neoplasm, and #2 is suspect malignancy although I'm missing a few of the other words, so am not as certain as to the full meaning of #2."

I was sitting on the floor of our living room as I read it. Cancer. I allowed a few tears to sneak out as I realized that there was something malignant inside my body. The doctors said it was 75% likely that these nodules were going to be malignant and advised a full thyroidectomy. But everything I had found online was saying that thyroid cancer is the most mis-diagnosed cancer as it's impossible to know, with 100% accuracy, if it's malignant until after the surgery is done. A longtime family friend of ours is a general surgeon who does a decent amount of thyroidectomies and he graciously corresponded with us via email regarding our next steps. He confirmed our research that even though the biopsy said suspicious for malignancy, it was 'unlikely' to be cancer but he'd have his pathologist take a look at it.

On a 'nudging' or whim, I looked up a large teaching hospital in our home State to see if they had an endocrine specialist and of course, they did. I spontaneously called him, from Turkey, and explained my situation and if he'd consult with me. While many doctors at highly respected institutions had very strict protocol as to what they'd offer prior to an in-person meeting, this kind and compassionate doctor agreed to a phone consultation with me if I'd send him all of my medical records. I did. He said that the biopsy report gave me a 90% malignancy risk and advised a full thyroidectomy. Our doctor friend on the other side of the state along with his pathologist put my risk at 10% and advised a 'watching and waiting' or at most, a partial thyroidectomy. I was confused and lacked a sense of peace as to what my next steps should be. Fortunately, we were flying home the next day and had made in-person appointments with both doctors as well as having the pathologist at the University of Michigan provide a second official pathology report.

Both doctors that I had consulted seemed to think that if anything, I had papillary thyroid cancer. In fact, the doctor at this university said that I was the 'classic' papillary thyroid cancer patient. I was still wavering on whether to even have surgery, as I didn't want this essential part of my body removed only to find out that it didn't need to be removed at all. So while this doctor was telling me this, I was still questioning everything and trying to make sense of it all. As we were leaving the appointment at the university, our doctor said that he wanted just a few more blood tests done to check my calcitonin and CEA levels. I joked with the lab tech as he took yet another sample of blood from my body. I had half-heartedly scheduled surgery at the university with the caveat that I might still opt for the unadvised partial thyroidectomy.

We were driving through the beautiful fields of Indiana when my endocrine surgeon called me. *Christen, your blood work came back.* He told me what numbers they like to see in normal, healthy patients and then said that my calcitonin level was measuring at 624 and my CEA was at 5. "What this means," he continued, "is that you have Medullary Thyroid Cancer…" I was trying my best to listen but the information was being absorbed in small doses. *"It could be familial but it's most likely sporadic, meaning you're just unlucky. But you may have to have your kids tested…The course of action is still the same, to move forward with a full thyroidectomy and central dissection that following week."* I heard two things from that confirmation. I had cancer, the less treatable and more rare kind. And, my kids might have it if I and they test positive for the genetic mutation of this cancer." How did I go from feeling like it was unlikely that it'd be cancer at all to having a confirmed kind of cancer that was more rare, less treatable, and possibly genetic?

One thing that I've learned from other people's stories with cancer is that you have to expect the unexpected. Cancer doesn't follow rules and sometimes it's the most unlikely outcome that comes to fruition. I went from thinking that I 'might' have a very treatable papillary thyroid cancer, if it's cancer at all, to one that wasn't leaving me with the same sense of optimism.

The heaviness of an unlikely diagnosis hits you at unexpected times. I remember my kids playing on a playground, I was lying down and looking at the big blue sky and all of a sudden, my husband looks over to find me sobbing while curled up in the fetal position. I had held it together for 6 weeks since the original nodule discovery. My 3-year-old son ran over to me and said, "Mama, are you sad?" "Yes, Sam. But I'm okay." He ran back to the slide and I allowed myself to cry.

I needed answers. I needed more information. Fortunately, a friend who had thyroid cancer had sent me the website for ThyCa and it was through that site that I connected with the "Meddie community". I'm not sure whether to be grateful for that or not. ☺ Sometimes, ignorance is bliss…. But other times, ignorance can kill you. I stumbled upon this community of people who were all in various stages of MTC. As I shared my story, they all were telling me to cancel my surgery and go to a Center of Excellence. Their stories and advice was unraveling me at the seams and again, leaving me with more doubts and uncertainty about who to trust for my care. Compared to many places around the world, a highly respected teaching and research hospital *is* considered an amazing place for care. But I was being told it wasn't good enough. But as I frantically sought second opinions from some of these experts, I kept coming up with dead ends. No one would take my case in a short amount of time. They were booked for several months. One assistant to one of these recommended experts accused me of doctor shopping! I tried to explain, "No, I just want more information. I just want more answers", but she wouldn't even connect me with the doctor or put me on his schedule. She seemed offended. I had cancer and I was scared. Unlimited time and resources was not something I had.

I asked those I trusted about this decision and as we all prayed about it, they all confirmed that they felt like this university was a great place for care. And they reminded me of how this surgeon was the only one willing to consult with me while I was thousands of miles away from my comfort zone. Sometimes it's an expert's availability and accessibility that can make all the difference in the world for someone's future. I decided to move forward with my scheduled surgery because my husband also had an upcoming foot surgery that needed to get done. I already felt like this cancer had greatly inconvenienced my life.

The night before my surgery, I did not feel settled. It felt too rushed. It felt too soon. It was just 6 days since I had found out I had Medullary Thyroid Cancer. I prayed for a natural way out or confirmation that I needed to have a few more weeks. The answer came at 2 am when I woke up to my son vomiting all over his bed. I scooped him up as vomit covered my pre-surgery body. A few minutes later, my GI bug symptoms started. There was no way I could move forward with surgery with this GI bug. I emailed my doctor at 4 am explaining the situation and called the hospital first thing in the morning. No go. What an upheaval of emotions to call it off… but I felt relieved, in between my bathroom trips, of course. The next available date was two weeks out. Surely that was enough time to get another opinion. After the dust settled, I started calling and getting information to MD Anderson and another expert in St. Louis. I was overwhelmed and frantically grappling for answers. MD Anderson quickly was acquiring all of my medical information and preparing an appointment for me. July 6 with Dr. Clayman. My current surgery date at the university was June 24. I have two small children, and a husband who needs two surgeries within the next month. I felt the weight of it all… How do I reconcile my desire to get the best care possible with the needs of my family? I tried to have my university surgeon consult with Dr. Clayman for my own peace of mind as to his approach to this first and most important surgery. He wouldn't do it. He flat out refused. He said that he knew Dr. Clayman and he would approach surgery the same way that he would. Well, who was I to question that? I was still going to a very great hospital with a specialist in endocrine surgery. Everyone I talked to, who hadn't received the wisdom of other "Meddies," felt like this university *was* great care. And it was. It was good… but I couldn't shake the feeling: "Was it good *enough*?"

Ultimately, I felt constricted by our life situation and knew that everyone else wanted me to stick with the June 24 surgery. So I did. But

I think this highlights the need for caregiver education and patient empowerment. I just needed one advocate to say: "Yep, cancel and go to the best of the best." I was the most researched on the cancer out of anyone in my immediate family and with a history of being more of a worrier – I didn't have a lot of street cred when it came to asserting that maybe I needed to go to a center of excellence. This will probably be something that comes back to me for the rest of my life. I had surgery a week ago. My incision is healing. My appointment with Dr. Clayman is still going to happen pending no cancellations on their end. I need more information and peace of mind. I don't have time to waste worrying about whether my care is good enough.

My pathology report from surgery came back yesterday. Yes, it was Medullary Thyroid Cancer. Yes, it had spread to my lymph nodes. Yes, I am now a Stage III MTC patient. I have my initiation scar as well as the anxiety that comes with this cancer. But I also have faith and peace knowing that my life is in the hands of my Creator. I have an overwhelming amount of support from family and friends. I have a husband who has been with me every step of the way and children who remind me that there is joy even while having cancer. I have made a commitment not to be defined by Medullary Thyroid Cancer, no matter how much it shapes me. I want to *be well*. I also want to lean into the wisdom of the MTC community as well as add joy and encouragement to it.

I'm a rookie. This is really fresh. The verdict is still out on the effectiveness of my first surgery. I don't know if this has spread elsewhere. I don't know how many years of stability that I will have. But here's what I do know: God knows the number of my days. He will make me well if I allow Him too. There are experts out there who can give me peace of mind knowing that I can do everything within my control to stay on top of this cancer. And finally, Cancer sucks… especially the rare, underfunded kinds that take everyone by surprise.

I'm going to MD Anderson in three days. I'm going to meet with a superhero, so I'm told by other Meddies. And I'm hoping to come away from that appointment with more confidence and understanding in what I am up against. I'm going to fight for the best care possible so I can care for my young children as long as possible.

Hi. I'm Christen. I'm 32 years old. I'm married to my college sweetheart. I'm a mom of two little, beautiful children. I'm a photographer and social worker. I live overseas. I have Medullary Thyroid Cancer, Stage III. I'm not a victim. I am more than a conqueror in Christ Jesus. I want to *be well*.

Dear Cancer

By Megan Morrow Bozeman

Dear Cancer,

You've been in my life for 4 years now. I know you don't plan on leaving me anytime soon. But you must know that as much as I want you gone, I also know that I may die because of you. As much as you get in my way every day, I *am* stronger than you. As much as you try to bring me down, I will *always* rise above you. Because of you, I have become spiritually stronger, and I thank you for that. When the day comes that you take my life, just know that I *never* lived with you, you lived with me. And despite all the heartache you put my family and me through, I will *always* be stronger than you.

You might take my life but you never touched my Spirit!

Megan